Experiences of Donor Conception

of related interest:

Looking for Oliver
A Mother's Search for the Son she Gave Up for Adoption
Marianne Hancock
ISBN 1 84310 142 4

Birth Fathers and their Adoption Experiences
Gary Clapton
ISBN 1 84310 012 6

The Adoption Experience
Families Who Give Children a Second Chance
Ann Morris
ISBN 1 85302 783 9

The Dynamics of Adoption
Social and Personal Perspectives
Edited by Amal Treacher and Ilan Katz
ISBN 1 85302 782 0

Lesbian and Gay Fostering and Adoption
Extraordinary Yet Ordinary
Edited by Stephen Hicks and Janet McDermott
ISBN 1 85302 600 X

Counsellors in Health Settings
Edited by Kim Etherington
ISBN 1 85302 938 6

First Steps in Parenting the Child Who Hurts
Tiddlers and Toddlers Second Edition
Caroline Archer
ISBN 1 85302 801 0

Next Steps in Parenting the Child Who Hurts
Tykes and Teens
Caroline Archer
ISBN 1 85302 802 9

Experiences of Donor Conception

Parents, Offspring and Donors through the Years

Caroline Lorbach

Foreword by Eric Blyth

Jessica Kingsley Publishers
London and Philadelphia

The right of Caroline Lorbach to be identified as author of this work has been asserted by her in accordance with the Copyright, Designs and Patents Act 1988.

First published in the United Kingdom in 2003
by Jessica Kingsley Publishers Ltd
116 Pentonville Road
London N1 9JB, England
and
325 Chestnut Street
Philadelphia, PA 19106, USA

www.jkp.com

Copyright © 2003 Caroline Lorbach

Library of Congress Cataloging in Publication Data
A CIP catalog record for this book is available from the Library of Congress

British Library Cataloguing in Publication Data
A CIP catalogue record for this book is available from the British Library

ISBN 1 84310 122 X

Printed and Bound in Great Britain by
Athenaeum Press, Gateshead, Tyne and Wear

Contents

A very brief look at the history of infertility treatment. An
explanation of the terminology used to describe the people
involved in donor conception.

Why is it still such a secret topic? How do infertile men feel,
how do they come to terms with not being able to have their
own biological child? How do these men's wives and partners
cope with the news of infertility?

How do women cope with not being able to conceive naturally
or to have their own biological child? Is their way of coping
different to men's?

What are the issues to look at when making the decision to use
donated gametes? How important is counseling in the
decision-making process? How do single women and
same-sex couples decide?

To Patrice for your understanding.
To my three children, Andrew, Callum and Elizabeth,
this book is for you.

Acknowledgements

My gratitude to all those people who entrusted me with their personal stories for use in this book. Considering how secretive donor conception has been for so long it is wonderful to note that of the ninety-four people who have been quoted in this book sixty-eight have asked me to use their real names. Thanks especially to Leonie, the world's best networker who put me in touch with so many people, and finally to my brother Paul for saying four little words he probably doesn't even remember: 'You can do it.'

"He knows the world and does not know himself."
Jean de la Fontaine (1621–1695)

Foreword

In early 1993 a small group met in Sydney to share their experiences of assisted conception treatment using donated sperm or eggs and of parenting children conceived following donor insemination. Initially calling themselves the Donor Insemination Support Group, this group subsequently embraced donor conception more comprehensively and became the Donor Conception Support Group of Australia (DCSG). Publication of *Experiences of Donor Conception*, written by Caroline Lorbach, one of the people attending that first meeting, is a fitting ten-year anniversary testimony to the pioneering work of Lorbach and her colleagues in the DCSG, not only in Australia, but also globally. In the decade since 1993, the DCSG has been one of the world's foremost (probably the foremost) campaign groups lobbying for donor conception to shed its ambiguous image, to abandon its preoccupation with secrecy and anonymity and to ensure that donor conceived people are no longer misled about their origins or denied information about their genetic heritage.

In pursuit of these objectives in 1997 Lorbach and others in the DCSG wrote and published a ground-breaking book entitled *Let the Offspring Speak*. While this book included contributions from academic researchers, policy makers and professionals involved in the provision of donor conception services, its greatest strength was that, for the first time to my knowledge, it brought together in a systematic way first-hand accounts of people who were personally involved in donor conception – parents of donor-conceived people, donors and donor conceived people.

Lorbach, currently the DCSG's consumer advocate, has drawn on the strengths of *Let the Offspring Speak* in *Experiences of Donor Conception*. Dispensing with the professionals (after all we get plenty of other opportunities to have our say), she provides a brief overview of male and female fertility difficulties, and then takes the reader through the stages of initial thinking about donor conception, through treatment, into the realms of parenting a donor-conceived child and the experience of being a donor-conceived child, young person or adult.

Lorbach draws on her own experience as the mother of three donor-conceived children and the experiences of other members of her family. She also draws extensively on the personal accounts of other parents, donor-conceived children, young people and adults, and of donors. The geographical spread of the accounts illustrated in the pages of the book is wide-ranging, including Australia, Canada, Germany, New Zealand, the UK and the USA.

What is especially impressive about this book is that Caroline Lorbach has sufficient confidence in her own editorial abilities to apply a relatively light touch. While her editorial hand is evident in the book's skilful structuring and sheer readability, it does not encroach on the personal accounts of her contributors.

Experiences of Donor Conception is an important contribution to contemporary debates on assisted conception services providing unique perspectives from donors, parents of donor-conceived children and donor-conceived people. It should be recommended to anyone contemplating becoming a donor or undergoing assisted conception services involving donated gametes. Existing donors, parents of donor-conceived children and donor-conceived people will also find much in here that resonates with and validates their own experiences. Last, but by no means least, this book should be compulsory reading for all those who provide donor conception services, regulators of donor conception services and legislators.

Eric Blyth BA MA PhD CQSW
Professor of Social Work,
University of Huddersfield

Introduction

What is there in life, in growing up, that prepares us for infertility? Nothing at all prepared me for infertility, neither my own nor my partner's. In my teens my mother talked to me about conception and the talk was laced with dire warnings of, 'Now, you won't get pregnant before you get married, will you?'

Being in my teens and early twenties in the 1970s meant I was, like everyone else, surrounded by talk of 'the pill' which was just becoming freely available. The media was full of articles about 'the pill' and what it meant for women; it seemed like the worries of teenage pregnancy and unwanted children were gone.

After I met my husband and we began living together, I religiously took the pill. That warning from my mother about not getting pregnant before I got married still rang in my ears. Little did I know that we weren't preventing anything. There was nothing to prevent: he had no sperm, and I rarely ovulated.

Through the ages, people have accepted infertility as a curse or, conversely, some have accepted it as a gift, giving them free reign. There have been many ways of circumventing infertility: adopting a child from another family; accepting the child of a brother or sister as one's own. Women have had sexual relations with a man other than their husband (usually unbeknownst to the husband), in order to hide their husband's infertility; men have also brought home children conceived by them with a mistress.

The late twentieth century abounded with hope for infertile people. The lead up to the birth of the first in vitro fertilization (IVF) baby in 1978 was full of promise; now infertility would finally be 'cured.' No one would ever have to feel the pain of longing for a child they could not have.

IVF and its related technologies have indeed enabled many thousands of people to conceive a much-wanted child, but what of those people who do not produce eggs or sperm, or those who fear passing on a genetic disease to a child – what is there for them?

Sperm donation has been around for a lot longer than most people realize, at least since the end of the nineteenth century when the first recorded use of donated sperm occurred. In 1884, Dr William Pancoast, a professor in Philadelphia, USA had been treating a woman who was unable to become pregnant. He eventually discovered that she was most likely fertile but that her husband appeared to be producing no sperm. He decided an 'operation' would be carried out on the woman to try to achieve a pregnancy. The woman was anaesthetized with chloroform and inseminated with the sperm of another man. There is no record of who the donor was – perhaps a medical student, perhaps Pancoast himself. The woman was never told what had been done to her, but nine months later she gave birth to a son.

Since the end of the nineteenth century, donor insemination has continued to be used by private doctors in many countries. From the beginning of the century up until the 1940s there were very few reports of artificial insemination by donor (AID) in medical literature, so we have no idea how many women may have given birth following the use of donated sperm. In the United Kingdom and Australia, AID began to be more widely used from the 1940s on. One report in an American medical journal of the 1940s suggested that there had already been nearly 9500 pregnancies in the USA using AID.

The estimates that are given on the number of children born from donor conception in any country are probably lower than the true figures because of the secrecy that has surrounded this form of assisted reproduction. Figures relating to frequency of use of donor conception are not often reported in most countries. Little consideration has been given to reporting the frequency of use in most countries – in fact it has been suggested that the reverse is true – great thought has been given to not reporting the figures.

For a long time we have been able to circumvent male infertility by using the sperm of another man, but nothing could be done if a woman produced no eggs, or eggs of such poor quality that conception was not possible. Since the first IVF birth in the late 1970s, it became possible for one woman to donate her eggs to another. The most common way for this to occur in the early days was for a woman already undergoing IVF to donate any eggs she did not use in a cycle. However, it was not until 1983 that the first baby was born as a result of a donated egg.

Sperm was successfully frozen as early as the 1950s and eventually the methods used for sperm were adapted for the freezing of embryos. This enabled couples to freeze spare embryos created during one cycle and use them in another. It also made possible the donating of embryos to couples who both had fertility problems or to a couple who could not obtain donor eggs. Although it is possible to freeze eggs, the viability rate after thawing is extremely low.

In the 1990s, the latest technique to aid infertile men has been intracytoplasmic injection (ICSI) where a single sperm is injected into an egg to achieve fertilization. ICSI is used in instances where a man has an extremely low sperm count or has motility problems (sperm which do not move well). This procedure is still expensive and some have had doubts about it because of the possibility of passing on genetic forms of infertility.

My husband, Patrice, and I are an infertile couple, and the fact that I have given birth to three wonderful children did not cure our infertility. Andrew (born 1989), Callum (born 1992) and Elizabeth (born 1995) were all conceived with the help of three men we have never met, three men who were sperm donors.

My understanding of donor conception and what it means for families did not really begin until Andrew was nearly four and Callum was a few months old. It began in a small but important way in 1993 at the meeting of 11 couples in Sydney, Australia one summer afternoon. All these couples either had children born by donor insemination or were trying to start their families by means of donated sperm or eggs. We talked until one in the morning, sharing our experiences. Most had never met another person who had used donor conception. Even though there was an underlying seriousness in our discussions, we still had time to laugh; one of the first suggestions for a name for our fledgling group was 'The Wounded Willies.'

Through the group I have met people involved in the area of donor conception worldwide and I have come to realize that people are desperate for any information they can get to aid them in their journey with donor conception. I have found that what people most want is to hear the experiences of others who have gone down similar paths, and that is why I put this book together. I have felt privileged that so many people, some of whom I have never met beyond emails, have entrusted me with their stories. One of the adults born of donor conception whom I interviewed for this book said a very wise thing that would be good to bear in mind when reading this book. She said that her views when talking to me might not always remain her views, that her thoughts where ever-evolving and I am sure that is true for all of us.

Terminology

The terms used for medical techniques and for the people involved in the area of donor conception have been evolving over decades. Originally, in male infertility, the term artificial insemination by donor (AID) was used, but in the 1980s, when acquired immune deficiency syndrome (AIDS) became well known, most people thought that the two acronyms were uncomfortably close and so we began to use the term donor insemination (DI). However, even before this there were some people (mostly parents) advocating a change to the term DI because they wanted to drop the word 'artificial.' The naming of methods of conception is still evolving as Christina describes. "We honestly haven't spoken about all the specifics of how and when we will tell our child/children about AI (alternative insemination…which is another way that is being used to describe the insemination process)."

What about the people involved in donor conception – what do we call them? Here are some of the terms I have heard over the years:

donor, provider, supplier

biological father/mother

natural father/mother

social father/mother/parents

recipient parents

Dad/Daddy, Mum/Mummy

donor offspring, DI adoptee, person born of donor conception, donor-conceived adult.

This list is by no means exhaustive. You will read many if not all of these words and phrases throughout this book. I don't support any particular ones over any others. Nancy explains how she feels about one term.

> It is with less acceptance however that I have noted the use of the term 'social parents' used in various media and press articles relating to IVF families. From my perspective, given that my body nurtured my child's growth for nine months and gave birth to this wonderful miracle, given that we love her unconditionally, and given that we are physically, emotionally, and legally responsible for her life, our attachment to our child constitutes much more than 'social parenting.' I hope that as more 'special' families are created and our profile increases, society will gain a greater understanding and respect for our individual situations.

In our family we use 'Dad' and 'Mum' for Patrice and me, and we talk about the men who provided the sperm as the 'donors.' Andrew has asked what the name of his donor is and I think if we knew the names of our children's donors then we would use them. I feel that each family has to find the terminology that is comfortable for them.

> Irene talks about the words they use in their family.

> The other thing I'd like to mention is the issue of comfortable terminology. This is a tough one, as we all have different comfort levels and our own personal feelings as to what a name means to us. We are using donor, or sperm donor, and it's OK for now. We use Dad, Daddy and Father for my husband. "Father" (used for the donor) would not be a choice I would be comfortable with for our family. Perhaps "donor father" would be more comfortable when they are older, I don't know, but I know that this is something we'll be talking about with them as we grow together as a family.

Priscilla, who is in her twenties, comments on the use of the term 'donor offspring'; one that is often used to describe people like herself who were conceived by donor insemination.

> It doesn't really bother me, I think what else could you say? I don't see myself as an adoptee, but offspring doesn't really seem right either, maybe DI person.

And one last comment from Rob.

> Look, they're just terms, words. In the end it's what's in your heart, what the feelings are, what the sentiments are, if you're doing the right thing and you're doing it from the heart you can't go too far wrong.

1

Male Infertility

I always imagined that in an infertile male you'd see it, it would be visual, he'd be a skinny little runt, a sick looking person but not so. (Julian, infertile and father of two DI sons)

Male infertility is a subject that seems to scare men. I remember my husband coming home after a Christmas party at work. He had been sitting at a table with a few men, including his boss who mentioned that he had seen Patrice's photo in the newspaper. Patrice told everyone around the table that he had been interviewed about his infertility. At that point his boss said 'Oh' and left the table. No one else seemed keen on talking about the subject except one man who muttered, 'I wouldn't wish something that bad on anyone.'

How many of us have met an infertile man? Most would answer 'never', but can we be sure? It is a subject that is still hidden away and one that people rarely talk about. Why do people shy away from talking about male infertility? The answer is not a simple one; it is closely tied up with mens' image of themselves and societies image of men. One answer may lie in the physical differences between men and women. In a woman the ovaries that provide her ability to conceive children are never seen, release of an egg is not visible. However, in a man, just about everything is in the open. Because of this, sex and fertility are in many minds inextricably linked. It can be difficult to separate a man's ability to conceive children from his ability to have sexual intercourse. All over the world people seem to closely connect male fertility to virility; conceiving a child is considered by many to be proof of manhood.

Why do people make jokes about men 'firing blanks' when no jokes are made about women not having eggs? The jokes about male infertility usually tend to be told by men. Maybe they don't want to accept that infertility is something that can happen to anyone so they make light of it. But then again, even some women seem to have a problem with male infertility; there is a feeling that men need protection from talking or even thinking about it.

Infertility is in itself not a life-threatening condition, and when men discover that they are infertile their emotional reactions can vary tremendously. For some it is a hurdle to overcome before they can realize their dreams of fatherhood. For others the news can be devastating, as it was for Ralf. 'When I got my first diagnosis, I fell into a deep black hole, because I realized what that meant to me and Claudia. We could never have a child together in the biological sense.'

Others have expressed similar feelings:

> I am 100% sterile and infertile…as a male the initial shock of being diagnosed as infertile was like a jolt of lightening hitting my body. I was completely devastated. To some degree I still am, however there is nothing I can do. (Peter)

> I couldn't believe it, I thought it could be a mistake, something wrong with the test. (Julian)

> I always wanted to have my own kids, I was thinking that I was going to grow old and lonely. (Paul)

> Well, I felt that it was the end of the world, I couldn't talk to anybody, I didn't want to talk to anybody, I kept it all bottled up. (Laurie)

It can be extremely difficult for couples having difficulties in conceiving to talk about the issue.

> After a year of trying to have a baby Gillian finally sat me down and said, 'We have to talk about this.' To be perfectly honest it had passed through my mind that one of us might have a problem but I hadn't dwelt on it, I kept hoping that we would conceive so that I didn't have to think about it. (Mark)

Another couple, Michael and Vivianne, had been trying to conceive for some time. Michael knew how worried Vivianne was about it so he decided to go for a sperm test.

We'd been trying for some time and I decided to take the matter into my own hands. I didn't tell Vivianne at the time that I went to see the doctor. You hear things all the time, it's always on the woman's side but I knew it could be her or it could be me. I went for a test and they said to bring a sperm sample. The result was hard to believe because I have a brother in France and he's a father; so I went a second time, I needed a second opinion. They told me the sperm count was zilch, zero. I went home and said, 'Look, Vivianne, I need to talk to you, stop worrying, I'm the one who's at fault.' I don't know the reason, it could have been a serious case of mumps, or I could have been born with something. The strange part of it is for her to have been on the pill for so many years and then find out I've been shooting blanks. For me, I could cope; it was watching Vivianne, denying her children. Watching someone else go through this, that was the difficult part.

The decision to undergo medical investigations may come after years of trying to conceive, as in Richard's case.

We were married in December 1984 and decided, as many newly-weds do, to hold off starting a family until we had the house and garden set up safely for children. We briefly tried for a baby in 1988, but with long service leave coming up in 1989 we decided to wait again. Heather did not want to become pregnant and be traveling overseas as well. We thought the romantic settings of Europe such as Paris or Rome might relax us enough for our family to begin. We returned after a wonderful three-month holiday but with no success. By late 1989, we had been having sex without precautions for over a year. Heather felt there might be a problem so she went along to the family doctor for a checkup.

However, the doctor suggested we both be tested to rule out any problems on either side. I felt a little concerned, but not overly so. If there was a problem, I felt sure that in this day and age it could easily be sorted out.

The doctor requested a semen sample that came back as low – less than one million sperm. I was referred to a urologist who found, on examination, a varicocele in my left testis. He suggested they tie off the blood vessels that were interfering with the sperm production and assured me it was a simple day surgery. Good results had been achieved in the past in raising sperm levels like mine to six million.

I was self-conscious of the procedure. I told no one at work about it, and only rang my supervisor after it was over, to inform her I was in hospital for a small operation of a private nature. I was worried people would find out about the problem. After all, this operation would fix it so there would be no need to inform anyone.

Our doctor referred us to a professor at W. Hospital. He ordered more tests and after the results came back, our options were limited to DI. The sperm test showed less than 300,000 viable sperm, or less than one percent chance of conceiving naturally.

While talk of female infertility has become more common in the media since the first IVF birth in 1978, male infertility, even though it accounts for approximately 50 percent of fertility problems, does not get the same coverage. This non-exposure must add to the feelings of isolation that many men (and couples) feel when faced with male infertility.

> We read sometimes about infertility in newspapers but why should we be the 'victims'? We couldn't believe it and didn't want to believe it, so to be really sure I went to a second doctor and had a biopsy. When I got the final result it was not so hard as the first diagnosis because I had several months to deal with the problem. I am a rational person who looks into the future and not back. I think it was harder for Claudia than for me to get this diagnosis and to get it confirmed twice. (Ralf)

Some men know that they might become infertile because of medical treatments for cancer or other conditions. These days counseling usually goes hand in hand with such treatments and the risk of infertility is discussed. Men are usually given the opportunity to freeze their own sperm for possible future use. Unfortunately, many years ago this was not always an option.

> I had actually had a kidney transplant about twenty-two years ago and we always had a feeling I might be infertile because of the medication I was put on. So we were kind of prepared for it, but even when we did get the news it was quite disheartening. (Rob)

Tim discovered he had cancer at a young age, an age when illness and fertility are not usually top of the list for a person to be thinking about.

> I had cancer, teratoma of the testes, when I was nineteen. I'd only ever had the one testicle and it basically had enlarged. I thought it was a sporting injury and had gone off to a GP at a medical centre, he sort of thought the same thing and didn't think much of it. Then I woke up one

night and the pain was unbearable. Still thinking it was a sporting injury I headed off to a sports clinic. They had one look at it and sent me across the road to a hospital. They did a biopsy on it and then took it out the next day. It all happened in a fair rush.

I suppose at the time I didn't think much about the infertility, it was more a question of getting on top of the cancer. Self-preservation more than self-promotion.

Tim admitted that not thinking in terms of marriage at the time did not encourage him to think long term about his infertility.

I suppose in terms of really feeling it, it wasn't until I was a fair bit older. Between twenty-one and my early thirties, to a certain extent, it was more a case of not thinking much of the consequences and taking advantage of the fact and having unprotected sex. It wasn't really an issue until I came down to thinking about getting married and having children that I thought, obviously, it's going to have to be a bit different.

Bob was married when he found out that he was infertile and the discovery had a profound effect on his marriage.

I was married in 1974, for eighteen months we tried to have children with no success. All the tests were done on the wife and she was fine so we made an appointment for me to go in and see our local doctor. It was a half-hour trip. We'd gone in, I'd donated some sperm and we'd gone walking around the town for two hours. We went back after the tests were done, walked into the doctor's office and were told just straight out, 'Mr Davis, you will never have children.' It really didn't make much sense at the time for the simple reason that that it was so to the point, there was no preamble. It wasn't, 'I've got some bad news for you...' There was no warning.

It really didn't sink in for six months but in that six months the wife decided that she wanted to be pregnant and had gone out with a number of other men in the area where I grew up. That created a situation in the marriage that ended it.

The break-up of his marriage and his infertility had a huge impact on Bob's life.

For the next five years, I went from someone who had a fair bit of common sense and intelligence to someone who really didn't care about what was going on. It didn't happen overnight, but in the same period of time I had a motor vehicle accident, then my father died and all those things combined put me into a suicidal frame of mind. There were even thoughts of having let my mother down because I couldn't provide the grandchildren that she wanted. I was in a frame of mind where I'd become what the Americans call a vagabond: I didn't live anywhere, I didn't take proper physical care. It was a very hard time emotionally, and as I started to come out of it in 1979 I turned it to my advantage, I used it as the greatest condom out.

A man who already knows that he is infertile when he enters into a relationship must decide at what point to tell a woman that he can never conceive his own biological children. When should this be done – at the first meeting, after you marry, when she decides that you should meet her parents, when you first sleep together – when? Bob chose to tell Glenda (now his wife) quite early on in their relationship.

I was working in Yass, she was working in Forster on the north coast, we'd written a couple of letters and I'd left the job in Yass and moved up to Forster. Sex in those days was a part of every relationship whether you were married or you weren't married. Once we started going out, I wanted to try and put her mind at rest about the possibility of causing her an embarrassment, so I told her I couldn't have children. It had the opposite effect – she thought I was pulling her leg and trying to become sexually involved more easily than through normal channels. It wasn't for quite a while that she came to even start believing it.

Acceptance of infertility is not always immediate. Some men, while they understand what their doctor is telling them, still live in hope that things might change, that all will be well and that the infertility might go away. My husband, Patrice felt like this.

In mid 1987 when we sat in the office of Caroline's gynaecologist and were given the blunt news that 'There are no sperm, the count is zero,' we were stunned. I don't recall any thoughts passing through my mind, it was blank. The doctor referred me to a urologist who performed a testicular biopsy. The result came back, a severe blockage, cause unknown and virtually no chance of surgically fixing it.

It's strange, we knew the cause of the problem, and it was very easy to understand why we couldn't conceive, but I still clung to the hope that perhaps they got it wrong. Maybe when I'd had the sperm test I'd been too nervous, that was why there was no sperm. Together Caroline and I collected a sample at home and I took it straight to the pathologist. Of course the result was the same, no sperm visible, there never would be.

Julian also took a while to come to terms with his first test results.

I was sure that the retest would show that I was fine. I couldn't believe it for a long time. Then when the retest came through and yes, I was infertile, I thought well, I can't be fully infertile, there must be a blockage, they'll clean that out and I'll be right. I just kept on thinking of ways out of it and just believed that underneath it I was fine and they'd fix me up. I knew nothing about male infertility, I thought it hardly ever happened, that it was very rare. I've never really got to the bottom of why I'm infertile. My two other brothers, they've both got kids, they've both had sperm counts and they're fine. One sister is married and has two kids.

There are men who have already had children in a previous relationship but then discover on entering a new relationship that they are now infertile. Their desire to have children with their new partner can be very strong and they can experience grief for the loss of the biological children that they and their partner thought that they would be able to have together.

David had two daughters and then had a vasectomy. After his first marriage broke up and he married Pam, they decided that they would like to have a child together.

When you have a vasectomy you've got to have a reversal within three years, mine was seven or eight. I went to the local GP and he sent me to a urologist. He was able to connect one testicle but he said the other didn't work. I had a very low sperm count, but then overnight I went from a count of five million motility to nothing.

The doctor, who hadn't done many vasectomy reversals, said there wasn't a great success rate. When we went to an infertility clinic we were sent to another urologist and he said that if he had done the operation he would have done it completely differently. He said I would have been confined to bed for so many days and on a very high course of vitamins, but after the operation I had been up and walking around almost as soon as the anaesthetic had worn off.

It is not unknown for men to offer their partner or wife a way out of the relationship when they discover that they cannot give them children.

I gave Leonie the option of getting out of the marriage. I originally thought she wanted to be married to someone she could have kids with. It must have made me feel like I wouldn't be a good husband. I don't think I felt that kids were an important part of marriage but I knew Leonie wanted to have kids; it was important to her to have a family. (Warren)

We had to wait six months for treatment with DI. During this time I came to the idea that my wife might decide to leave me for someone who could give her a family without all the hassle. I was feeling very low. My wife reassured me that this was not her idea, only mine, but the fear of rejection at this time was distressing for many weeks. (Richard)

Claudia, while trying to come to terms with the shocking news of her husband's infertility, was asked a very difficult question.

We married in 1993, one year later we noticed that something must be wrong. So we both went to our doctors. Ralf's urologist told us he has no sperm. He went to another doctor with the same result. We couldn't believe it. To be completely sure, Ralf went to hospital for a biopsy of the testicles, there was not one sperm in it. We were very disappointed and frustrated, our world broke down. It took a long time to handle it.

Ralf asked me if I would have married him if I had known about his infertility before. I answered that I didn't know. This answer was hard for Ralf, because he knew that I always wanted to have babies. But I never thought about leaving him.

Wendy's husband seemed to be expecting that his wife would leave him.

My husband was born without a vasdeferens. We didn't discover this until we had tried for a while for a child without success and then went for tests. When he came home that night, after receiving the results, he was devastated and asked if I was going to divorce him. I, of course, said no, and we began exploring options.

Women can react with shock when faced with the discovery that their partner is infertile. This is perfectly natural; it is hard to realize, while you may be perfectly capable of conceiving a child, your partner will never be able to do that. Vivianne found the initial discovery very difficult.

We were just getting very frustrated trying to conceive. I had a regular cycle. I was quite ignorant, I didn't know anything about infertility. I was getting very emotional about it, hoping that maybe one month we'll get it right. Michael was working seven days a week and I was working, I thought it was all stress related. Michael went and took the matter into his own hands before I actually reached that point of saying that maybe we should do something about it. When he told me his test results, that he was infertile, what flashed in front of me was total loss. This overwhelming, 'My God, I will never have my own child.' This was so major, everything up to now had been able to be fixed, this couldn't be fixed.

Janet also found it a shock.

We'd been married for about a year and a half and we started thinking about having a child, I already had some concerns about my fertility because I'd ovulated irregularly and had short cycles. I went to a local doctor, a woman who was fantastic. She suggested it would be easier to get us both in at once because testing Julian was much less intrusive. I had a blood test first and at the same time Julian had his sperm test. We were expecting that to be fine. I rang for the results a few days later and she said, 'Look, there could be some mistake but Julian has a complete lack of sperm.'

That's how we found out. We had a retest and there was nothing there at all. I actually didn't feel anything initially, a complete lack of feeling for a while. The reaction after that was disbelief because we felt in our ignorance that Julian would somehow look different if he was infertile. We imagined that an infertile man would be small and weedy looking and unwell. We couldn't believe it, it was a complete sense of disbelief that this incredibly healthy person could be infertile. I think shortly after that the grieving process started but we still hoped that there would be a reason for this, that there was a blockage and there was something that could be done to cure it.

We did a lot of reading, we went to the library and got books on male biology and were checking out diagrams and thinking, 'maybe this tube could be blocked.' We were trying to find possible reasons for ourselves and really hoping that somehow it would be OK. We then saw our first specialist he had a look at Julian and said that for a fellow his size his testicles were a little on the small side, although within the normal range. They weren't able to give us any reasons. They discussed the possibility of a blockage but there were no swellings so it probably wasn't that. We weren't left feeling satisfied because we didn't know why.

Nicky grieved the fact that they might never have a child of their own.

We had foolishly announced we wanted to start a family, so as time passed people began to ask. At first we felt too battered to tell anyone and made up stories about saving money first, but each time I lied my heart was just crying inside. I was grieving the chance to nurture a little baby and threw myself into nurturing lots of veggies and flowers in pots on our tiny terrace. My letters home were full of how many centimetres my lettuces or sunflowers had grown, but I wished it had been news of our baby. Holger grieved more for the passing of his genes but for me it was the nurturing, and the realization that the future as I'd always seen it was gone. For the first time in my life I realized we can't plan our lives.

Some people said I should be glad I was fertile. But I often wished the problem was in me and I could feel more in control of doing something about it. But my husband was infertile and the end result was the same – as a couple, we were and still are, infertile.

In the next six months or so, I fell into a deep depression. I kept asking 'Why us? It's not fair.' It was such a silent grief, I felt so alone. I felt I'd lost all control of my life, everything was black. I remember saying to my mum, 'I can't see where my life is heading' and she replied, 'You have to find a way.' It was a very frightening time. I'm normally an energetic, go get it type of girl, but wanted to just curl up in bed all day. No counseling was offered, just the attitude – get on with it. Not being able to have a child as expected struck the very core of my being. What was the point then? Where was the future now? I'd never wanted to be a real career woman but maybe I'd have to now. All around me, women fell pregnant, often accidentally. Every Christmas card in 1996 contained news of a new pregnancy or photos of a new baby.

I just couldn't deal with it. The hardest blow was when my younger sister, who had never been clucky, announced her pregnancy. That affected our relationship for a long time – my pain and her unnecessary but natural guilt were too much. I lost all sense of self. Who was I now? With all the other changes in my life I just felt like the carpet had been pulled from under my feet.

How men and women find out about their infertility can make a huge difference to their ability to cope with the news. While the vast majority of doctors handle the passing on of information about infertility with compassion and understanding, there have been times when people have found out in very harsh ways.

> Ken had a couple of tests; he had a sperm test first, which identified a problem, then the testicular biopsy confirmed that there was no sperm production. The way he was told wasn't terribly good – the doctor just rattled off the bad news, closed the book and said, 'I'm going on holidays.' (Rose)

Joanne and Greg had fertility tests done before they were married because they knew that Greg might have problems, but the results were a long time coming.

> When Greg was twenty he had Hodgkin's disease and had chemotherapy. Before we were married we decided to have a fertility test. I was twenty and Greg was twenty-five. Greg gave a sperm sample at his GP's. We didn't hear any more. About six months after we were married Greg went to see his oncologist (he was still having regular check-ups) who told Greg, 'I'm sorry about the results of your sperm count.' Greg asked, 'What do you mean?' The specialist told Greg, 'You're sterile.' Greg came home and told me. It was a shock. I rang the GP's surgery next day from work and asked if there was a letter that came back with the test results. I was told, 'Yes, I'm really sorry you weren't told.' I was absolutely shattered that they all knew about this before we did and that the GP had never contacted us. Apparently he did say to Greg's mother that he didn't think it was a good idea that we got married. Greg's mother, at the time, thought that Greg had come out of remission.
>
> That was how we found out, that's why I'm not even forty yet and we've got a sixteen-year-old daughter and we're an infertile couple, that's absolutely amazing. So we were lucky in that sense. I'd hate to think that we could have been like so many others, worked for three or four years and then tried to fall pregnant for four years and then found out.

Bridget knew that Tim was infertile before they were married but she said that the true impact of this didn't hit until some time after their marriage.

> I've always wanted children, and in fact when Tim told me he was infertile I remember going to sleep that night thinking, 'It's such a shame, he's such a nice bloke but I'll wake up tomorrow and I won't be interested in him any more.'

> I was pretty gutted that he was infertile and my immediate reaction was, 'Oh, you'd obviously have to use your brother's sperm or something.' I probably didn't really face it until later on when things were getting pretty serious between us. I think I found the reality of it quite devastating. I didn't really face it until I had to. We had a terrible first year of marriage because we were having to deal with difficult issues in a relatively new relationship. I thought love could conquer all and that it was no big deal but in fact it was.

Glenda's view was somewhat different. Bob had also told her before they were married that he was infertile, but after initial disbelief she accepted it very quickly.

> When Bob and I met and we decided to be together I said to him, 'I must go on the pill' and he said, 'No, you don't need to, I can't get you pregnant.' My response was, 'Oh, sure, that's what they all say.' Slowly we started talking and he told me that he found out during his first marriage when he was about twenty-four that he was infertile.
>
> And that is how I found out that he can't father children. It didn't mean anything at the time, it just meant that I didn't have to go on the pill. Most couples in these donor programs have gone through the denial, the rejection, the blame, the why me. I never went through that because Bob had already gone through it. He had quite a long time to come to the fact that he cannot father children and he did it without me.

The media regularly have stories about people unable to have babies; these articles just about always focus on the grief of the woman. It is as though a man is expected to have very little feeling about an inability to conceive. Belinda experienced this first hand.

> From some people, the support was there for me but not for Michael. A friend of ours, when we told him, pretty much said to Michael that it wasn't important and he would be crazy to worry about not being able to have kids. Shortly after, the same person was talking to me and was really kind and understanding. The impression I got was that it was acceptable for a woman to grieve over these things, but it was unmanly for a man to let it bother him.

Charlotte tried to understand how her husband was feeling and let him express those feelings.

I was very supportive of him, was very aware of what was going on with him, I was very anxious to do things in a way that wouldn't hurt him, it made no difference to the way I felt about him. I made a lot of effort to try and find out how he felt. I did initiate conversations when he, perhaps, didn't want to talk about it, ultimately it was a good thing. I also really urged him to tell people rather than keep it a secret, which ultimately was better for him.

2

Women's Infertility

The majority of us grow up expecting that one day we will have our own children. Even being in my early twenties when the first IVF birth hit the headlines didn't mean that I learnt anything much about infertility or even thought about it. I certainly didn't at that time understand how common infertility is and never expected that it would touch me in such a lifelong way. Many others have had similar thoughts.

> I took it for granted...I grew up in a generation where I'd finish studying, have a career, then stop and have a family, then go back to work. That's just how it would work.

My own trek of discovery began about a year after Patrice and I were married. Shortly after the wedding, I stopped taking the pill and we used condoms for a few months as I felt that I should let the pill get out of my system before conceiving a child. While in the past children had never been at the top of my list of priorities, I, like so many others, just assumed that when the time came and I wanted to have children it would happen. But it didn't. After a year, I still had not menstruated. I had never been regular in my cycles but never queried a doctor whether this could affect my chances of conception. I'd grown up reasonably healthy and never felt the need or the curiosity to find out much about the workings of the female body. At this stage I was getting on towards twenty-nine and Patrice was thirty-two. There wasn't a feeling that I was about to run headlong into the brick wall of 'being too old to conceive,' it was more a selfish feeling of 'it wasn't like this in my plans.'

> The expectation that a woman will have a child is not just an instinct within her to perpetuate the species but an expectation from society; it is her 'role.'

I thought, I'll never have a family, never have a child. I thought that there would always be something missing, I would never have fulfilled all my womanly roles. (Vivianne)

June's journey to motherhood began during her first marriage.

Just six weeks before I was due to get married I went into hospital to have my appendix out. After they took it out I still had all this severe pain, and ended up back in hospital. They discovered that in fact I had an infected fallopian tube, they had to operate again because I was so ill. They removed the tube, and the gynaecologist said that by the time they removed it, it was the size of his thumb, it was huge.

I had continual problems with ovarian cysts and was told by my gynaecologist, 'Really you should start a family straight away.' But we were young, and about a year later I ended up having the ovary on that same side removed. I knew that there was a potential that I might have problems getting pregnant, but no one sat down and explained what the impact of losing one ovary might have on my fertility.

While June's infertility began with the removal of an ovary, things did not end there.

Later, my first marriage broke up; we'd been together for about five years. I got on with having a career, went overseas and then later moved back to Perth. I met my husband, Graeme, it was a bit of a whirlwind romance, we both wanted to have a family and spend the rest of our lives together.

All this time I'd been on the pill, so I stopped taking it. When I'd been off the pill for about six weeks, I started getting about thirty hot flushes a day, and became very moody. I went to my GP and had a hormone profile done. My doctor rang me at work and left a message to say my results were in. I thought that if he'd rung me at work it was obviously good news so I didn't ring him until the next day. He told me over the phone while I was at work that I was menopausal. I was thirty-seven and I was horrified, destroyed. I hung up the phone and rang my girlfriend who works in the next suburb and burst into tears. I couldn't ring my husband because I knew he'd be in meetings, and it was a personal, female issue and I wasn't ready to tell him. I told my girlfriend that she'd have to come and get me. She came and provided a shoulder to cry on.

Menopause – change of life, call it what you will, for someone like June, still in her thirties, it must have felt like the end of life: something, at that moment, so intrinsically female that only another woman could possibly understand what she was going through.

Anne also went through premature menopause and found it a very isolating experience.

> We'd been overseas and decided it was time to start a family, but after ten months I wasn't pregnant. My husband Carl was coming back to Australia for a conference, I thought I would come back too and just make sure that there weren't any problems. He had a test done and that appeared to be normal and then a couple of days later I went in to have a laparoscopy. I had endometriosis. It was some years before we ended up in IVF.
>
> After the endometriosis was cleared up I was put on clomid and I had a lot of side effects from the danazol I was also on for the endometriosis. Ultimately my cycles never returned to normal. Blood tests identified various unusual hormone levels but nothing very concrete. We started off having AIH (artificial insemination by husband), which wasn't successful, and then I didn't respond all that well to stimulation procedures. Down the track it became apparent that I was going through menopause.
>
> No one else seemed to be in the same boat as I was. There was no one I could find who had experienced a premature menopause. If I went to a seminar on menopause, everyone was twenty years older than me. Everyone else on IVF seemed to have 'common' problems. The few women I heard of having donor egg treatment were doing so because of their age and I just couldn't relate to that, seeing my problem as a medical one and theirs a result of life choices.

Anne did eventually conceive on a donor program but as she says she is still infertile and the birth of a beautiful baby girl did not totally take away the pain.

> When talking about it the time scale tends to get lost. Being twenty-seven at the beginning of fertility treatment and forty at the 'end' also impacts on perspectives. I say 'end' euphemistically. There is no end to infertility, it will always be a part of me and the grief I felt at having a hysterectomy last year was not tempered by having a child any more than her birth cured my premature menopause. This, despite knowing that I would never be pregnant again anyway. There is nothing more final than a hysterectomy — even more final than the loss of my genetic child through menopause.

If a couple wanting a child do not conceive, who will people think has the problem? Will they assume it is the man or the woman? Or both of them? Not so long ago it was not unheard of to find that a husband had never undergone any fertility tests while his wife had been put through a barrage from simple blood tests to a laparoscopy under full anaesthetic.

My first appointment with a fertility specialist was not overly long and very businesslike. I was asked a great many questions about my medical history. The doctor started asking questions about my husband but these stopped as soon as I said that Patrice had two children from his first marriage. After the physical examination all the doctor could tell me was that I had no obvious problems, and he ordered blood tests plus a CAT scan of the pituitary gland. When I went back for the test results, I was told that the scan was all clear but that the blood tests showed that I had a 'hormone problem.' I had so many half-formed questions but I just didn't have the knowledge to ask any proper ones. All I managed to ask was, 'What causes the hormone problem?' The only answer I got was, 'You were probably born with it.' I was prescribed clomiphene to try and encourage ovulation.

At that moment when I knew we might have problems trying to conceive, the desire to have a child intensified dramatically. Maybe it's a part of human nature that if someone says 'no' to you, you want it all the more. I don't think that I could even have explained why I wanted children. I just did. I took clomiphene for months but with no success. We moved house at about this time and I changed specialists. My new specialist performed a laparoscopy on me, which was all clear. He then decided that Patrice should have a sperm count done and we found that both of us had fertility problems.

After this the feeling I had of wanting a child grew even more. I remember standing in the middle of my living room one day and feeling like the world was closing in on me. I had suddenly realized that maybe there would never be anyone to call me 'Mummy.'

Our journey to discover the answers to our failure to conceive and our beginning on a donor conception program lasted a number of years, but it was short and relatively easy compared to that of some others.

It took Kate and John many years to discover the cause of their infertility, but for them also an assumption was made that there was nothing wrong with John.

We had been married for two and a half years and had decided to go overseas on what we labeled 'the conception tour.' We wanted a 'made in Europe' child. Before going, we were sure that I would be returning to Australia pregnant, but nothing happened.

A few more months went past and I sensed that there was something wrong, I was getting more and more anxious about it so off I went to see the local doctor. Initially he said that it took the average couple up to twelve months to conceive, but I just sensed things weren't quite right. I know my body well and we were doing what we were supposed to be doing at the right time. At that stage, only six months had passed from when we initially started trying, but the doctor sensed that I was rather anxious and said, 'How about getting John in to do a semen analysis because it's much easier to cancel out the male factor and then we'll go on from there, but I'm sure we'll find everything's normal.'

When the semen analysis was done he called us in and said, 'I think I'd like John to do another test.' The second test revealed the same result, which was a much reduced sperm count, but more worrying was the lack of motility. I saw it initially as any other problem, let's solve it. John's reaction was quite different; he felt he was letting the side down. We went to see a urologist, John had a varicocele operation done which wasn't successful, and we had to wait a few months to ascertain that. We were then referred to an IVF specialist who told us that ICSI was our only option.

We had three ICSI attempts, which were not successful. The worrying thing was that we were getting plenty of eggs but the resulting embryos were fragmenting and were never good enough to freeze. After our third cycle they said perhaps it could be an egg problem as well. This was after three years of rather intensive treatment. So in order to see if that was the case we tried a GIFT procedure using donor sperm but the resulting embryos were basically the same. Then we had quite a few DI attempts, which also weren't successful. Our next step, seeing that our eggs and sperm weren't working together and seeing as donor sperm wasn't helping, was to go to donor embryo.

For some women not being able to experience pregnancy and birth is almost too awful to contemplate, as Leigh describes.

My sisters and my brother all have kids; I'm the baby of the family. Alan and I got married in our early twenties but went overseas for a couple of years, working and traveling.

When we got home and settled down we decided that we didn't want to wait too long to have kids. Two years later nothing had happened and the results of the tests said that I might never have children. It was terrible and is still sometimes so terrible that I try not to think about it too much.

Although we could probably adopt as we're still young I want to have a child that grows inside me. I've felt the babies kick in my sisters' stomachs, I want life that moves inside me too. Even though counseling has helped I still feel this huge need to have a child.

How do men cope with their partner's infertility? How do they handle such devastating emotions as those felt by Leigh. Men, it could be said, are one step removed from conception – it does not happen in their bodies. While IVF now means that conception is possible in a glass laboratory dish, the embryo will not continue to grow and be born until it implants itself in the uterus of a woman. There are very few opportunities for men to talk about the emotional impact of their partner's infertility. Many feel a sense of helplessness that there is little they can do. They can also feel a sense of isolation almost akin to infertile men.

I tried to talk to my brothers but they just couldn't understand. A lot of people expressed sympathy but they really couldn't comprehend. I think it was particularly so for Anne but I also didn't have anyone to talk to. Anne went through so much, I felt helpless. If at any stage she had said that she didn't want to do it I would have supported her. In fact a number of times I sat her down and said do you really want to keep going with this? (Carl)

When Leigh's doctor gave us the news that we might never have children because of Leigh's problem with producing eggs I immediately wanted to be able to fix things. I asked question after question, looking for a solution that didn't exist.

I went into a depressive state and wasn't a particularly nice person to be around. It took me a good many months before I could even talk properly to Leigh about it. She had needed me and I had hidden myself away. She finally told me that I had to go with her to counseling which I reluctantly did. It was the best thing that I could have done; I gradually came to accept that not everything can be 'fixed'. I came to understand that even though we might still go on to have a child, maybe through egg donation, I still had to grieve the child that would have been ours together. (Alan)

Many husbands and wives are together in a doctor's surgery when they get their fertility results, but as June described previously she was in her office by herself and was told over the telephone that she was pre-menopausal. After she told her girlfriend she still had to tell her partner.

> Then I had the issue of telling Graeme, he wanted a family as well so what would happen with us, was it the end of our relationship? He was great, he was extremely empathetic. He said, 'I want to be with you, yes I would love to have a family, but it's not like it's the end of our relationship.'

With the support of Graeme, June felt the need to regain some control over her life.

> I was very disappointed with my doctor's lack of empathy. When I went to see him and asked what I could do he said, 'No one will be able to help you, you'll just have to get on with your life and recognize that having children is not everything.' He didn't suggest counseling. I asked for a referral to my gynaecologist and he said, 'Well, she's not going to be able to do anything for you either,' and I said, 'Well I want to go and talk to her.' When I went to see my gynaecologist she was at the other end of the spectrum to my GP. 'Oh, look June, women have all these different things happening to their bodies, really the medical profession doesn't know that much about women's bodies and what's going on, I've got clients who go in and out of menopause.'
>
> I also went to see a naturopath. I felt like I had no control but the naturopath, she said, 'Here are some things you can do, you can change your lifestyle, food, start to meditate.' I stopped work and focussed all my attention on looking after my body in an attempt to fall pregnant. I meditated every morning, I stopped smoking and I didn't drink. It gave me a feeling of being able to do something.
>
> Graeme was extremely supportive and did a meditation course with me. I also went and had some additional counseling. I wasn't really in the grieving process; I was probably in denial.

While June now felt that she was doing something positive to achieve her goal. Things changed rapidly.

> At the end of November that year I fell pregnant naturally. We were ecstatic; it was a miracle for us but around New Year I started getting pains. I went to a GP and said, 'I'm really concerned, I've had these problems and lost a tube, could I have an ultrasound to see what's going

on?' He said, 'Well, no, but we can do that next time you come, we couldn't see anything at the moment.'

The pains worsened one night and we went to the women's hospital. I had an ultrasound there but they said that they needed better equipment and could I come back tomorrow? The next day I went in to have another ultrasound. I was lying there waiting for the doctor to come and I said to Graeme, 'The pains are getting bad.' They got just excruciating, screaming stuff. Graeme raced off, grabbed a doctor who came and examined me. He got the ultrasound machine and said, 'I'm sorry but you've got an ectopic pregnancy.' The pregnancy had settled in the stump that was left after they'd removed the tube, it was also settled on the corner of the uterus and it had ruptured the uterus. I had an emergency operation. I was very lucky I was in hospital at the time it happened. Afterwards I was devastated about losing my baby, but was determined to fall pregnant again.

When I came out of hospital Graeme had a contract to go overseas. The obstetrician who operated referred me on to someone in Singapore where we were to move for six months. Once my body settled down I went on to clomiphene, so in the time I was in Singapore I did ovulate once but didn't fall pregnant. When we moved back down here I went back to my naturopath who referred me to a GP who was doing quite a bit of work with natural progesterone cream in women who were menopausal. He said, 'One thing we'll have to do is we'll have to track you and see what's happening.' So I began having regular hormone profiles done and my hormones actually started to become more normal. He referred me to an IVF specialist who put me on a program to try and stimulate my ovaries.

The first IVF cycle I produced only one egg and we waited to see if it fertilized. Graeme's sperm was fine; it was really healthy, which was a plus for us. The day before Graeme and I got married we found out that the egg hadn't fertilized. The upside of that was we got to drink champagne at our wedding. It was bizarre to have these things happening in the background while everyone around us was saying, 'It's wonderful you're getting married.' After that I went back to the IVF program but my body didn't respond. My GP put me back on the natural progesterone cream and that helped control the mood swings. The IVF specialist didn't think that they could do anything unless I used donor embryos or donor eggs. At that point I thought I needed a break.

When a specialist can find no reason for a couple's inability to conceive it is labeled 'unexplained infertility.' Nancy's infertility was described as 'unexplained', but this only added to her frustration.

We unknowingly commenced a six-year trek down the IVF road. A trek my husband, with three adult children from his first marriage, did not relish but none the less selflessly supported. Six years made more frustrating by the fact that medical technology could overcome any physical problems involved but could not explain my continued lack of conception.

Anyone who has been in the situation of unexplained infertility will be able to relate, I'm sure. Each unsuccessful cycle brings with it varying degrees of disappointment, sadness, anger, frustration, bewilderment and grief. These emotions were often very strong and difficult to overcome. Similar emotions were also evoked through other experiences, whether it be an unwanted pregnancy resulting in termination by distant family members, or a young nephew curling his arm around his father's neck for reassurance. There were constant displays of the unattainable parenthood which I coveted. The poignancy of these everyday occurrences, like our IVF experiences, are probably impossible to convey successfully to any but the childless couple who do not want to be childless.

3

Making the Decision
to Use Donor Conception

Very early in their marriage Joanne and Greg knew that they would have fertility problems because of Greg's cancer treatment. They knew that Greg had no sperm. At the time, they thought that adoption was their only option.

> We ended up down in Sydney and spoke to a counselor at Youth and Community Services about adoption. She basically told us that Greg was too old. Greg was twenty-six and a half by that stage and we were too old for adoption.

When they found out almost by 'accident' of the existence of another possible solution to their childlessness it came as quite a surprise.

> We were at a friend's place playing cards one night, having a few drinks, feeling sorry for ourselves, and we told them about our infertility. Carol said, 'Well what about artificial insemination?' We'd never heard of it. She went on to say that she and Dave had a friend who had three children and one day she had turned to that friend and said, 'My God, your child looks just like you, I can't believe how much he's like you.' This man had replied, 'They're not my children, they're artificially inseminated children.'
>
> We went and saw a GP and asked him about it, and he referred us to a clinic. We were married in 1980 and I conceived Lauren in 1982. It was really quick, I don't think we had time to stop and think.

In the late 1980s, when Patrice and I were faced with our infertility, my gynaecologist gave us two options: 'You can either adopt or use artificial insemination.' After one quick phone call we found out, like Joanne and Greg, that adoption was not a choice as we were already getting too old. So here was our lifeline, artificial insemination.

The question must be asked whether we sat down and discussed the implications of using donor insemination as individuals or as a family ourselves and most particularly on any child that we might have. The very simple answer is, 'no'" All we wanted at that stage was a child, and for me especially it almost became an all-consuming passion. No one suggested to us that there might be more to donor conception than achieving a pregnancy or the birth of a much longed-for child.

The specialist at the infertility clinic told us that we would most likely be able to achieve a pregnancy using DI. The nurses all talked about 'achieving a pregnancy.' No one ever talked about a child or the adult he or she would grow into. Even when we told the specialist that if we had a child we would tell him or her how they were conceived all the doctor said was, 'No one else needs to know. You don't need to tell anyone how the child was conceived.' Did he mean that even the child did not need to know? Yes, I think he did.

We never saw a counselor, there was one at the clinic and the doctor said that if we wanted to see him we could. But we were traveling right across the other side of the city at incredibly early hours of the morning to go to this clinic and the counselor was only there on one day a week at 11am. Besides, why did we need to see a counselor? We were both happy about our decision to use DI. We both agreed about telling any child we had about their conception, what more did we need to discuss? Weren't counselors for people with problems? We'd never known anyone who'd been to see a counselor. The doctor never suggested that counseling could be a good thing, he never mentioned what might be discussed in a counseling session.

At that stage we had not met another person who was also using donor conception. We didn't know anyone who had children by donor conception. We just thought that achieving our child was the end of things. Even the decision to tell our child of their conception was to us a simple thing. We would tell them, we saw nothing more than that, the vision of our future ended there. It never occurred to us there might be something more that needed to be considered before we decided to go ahead with using donor sperm.

I wish that things had been different for us and thousands of others, like Anne, who conceived her child nearly twenty years ago. 'We came to the decision in isolation. There were no counselors available and we didn't feel we could discuss it with family or friends. It was very lonely.'

To have a child using donated gametes is not a decision to be taken lightly. The child's needs, their need to be loved, to know where they come from, may be no different from other children's but the parent's ability to satisfy some of those needs may well be different depending on what facilities are available for information sharing with the child's donor. Decision making in donor conception has changed through the years from a time when no counseling was available, secrecy was the norm and questions were not encouraged to a time now where prospective parents in a number of countries are actively encouraged to discuss with a counselor the long-term implications of using donated gametes before making a decision to go ahead. Indeed, in some countries, counseling is a compulsory part of a donor program for all concerned, prospective parents and donors.

How do parents who conceived long ago feel about the lack of counseling?

> We just simply went along with the whole scenario without asking any questions. I don't know whether it was that we didn't know what to ask. I was brought up that you didn't question authority and some of those authoritarian types are doctors and nurses. Therefore I didn't think that I should be asking questions and Glenda being fairly shy didn't do anything but follow my lead. That, now, is probably one of the biggest let-downs of the whole situation. I think it would have been very helpful if we'd had counseling as a part of the scenario. (Bob)

> Nothing seemed to matter a great deal then apart from getting couples pregnant. Where was their foresight? They must have known that this is a loaded gun. I don't hold anyone person personally responsible for this and I also acknowledge the fact that I signed a disclaimer that I wouldn't pursue any donor information but I don't think I knew what I was signing. But boy, oh boy, the thing that makes me angry as much as anything else was that we had virtually no counseling at all. We saw a counselor and basically because Greg thought it was a good idea to have DI in order to have children we were passed. (Joanne)

Evelyn and Laurie made the decision to use DI about thirty years ago, when it was almost a totally closed subject.

> It was a very lonely decision, Laurie was pretty comfortable but it felt an immoral decision, to a degree. You were brought up with really strict morals in those days; it seemed akin to adultery.

Vivianne and her husband had both been married before, but while Vivianne already had children her husband did not.

> We'd had miscarriages from natural pregnancies and my gynaecologist wanted to send us off to an infertility clinic. As I was over forty, I asked, 'Won't my age prevent me from being accepted?' The doctor said, 'You don't look your age so don't worry.'
>
> So I went on an IVF program. Every morning my husband was running me up to the clinic for injections over a period of about six weeks. One day I was called into the office and the clinic doctor said, 'What's the story exactly? Your body looks like it's not producing eggs.' I told him my age and he said, 'Oh well, that's not a problem, we can more or less guarantee you a pregnancy if you accept donor eggs.' The idea had not occurred to me before and it was all too 'high-tech.' I wept as I thought 'I can't do that.' The doctor reassured me that the donor would be matched as closely as possible to my characteristics, so my husband and I went home to think it over. My husband thought it was all OK, and after talking it over we rang the clinic and agreed to accept donor eggs. We were never given any counseling or asked if we wanted any, and at that time all we had in mind was a little, lovable, squirming baby. We didn't think of all the repercussions and everything involved later on, down the track.

From my own experiences and from talking to others I am a strong advocate for the need to have a properly informed discussion about all the implications of using donor conception before making a decision. I see a counselor as being the best person to help with this, but counseling also needs to be strongly supported by medical professionals in infertility clinics.

Janet conceived her first child about seven years ago at a clinic which provided counseling but, as she illustrates, counseling, while presenting the theory and an avenue for guided discussion, will not provide everything that prospective parents need.

The counselor helped us look at issues that we either hadn't thought about or hadn't wanted to look into more deeply, such as how the child would deal with it. It was never an issue for us to keep it a secret, right from the start we decided our children had that right to know. It's an enormous responsibility to think that you're creating a life in this way and you just want to be sure that you're equipped to help them deal with the implications of it. I used to feel quite guilty thinking that if this child isn't happy or goes through adolescence and has a difficult time with it I might feel that I'm somehow responsible for adding to that.

One of the other big issues was the lack of medical information, the possibility of the child developing a condition and not having the donor's medical history. I think it was a kind of selfishness in the end, that we needed to have children more. I think you justify it by saying, 'Well children are adopted and might not know their background and some other people don't have close relationships with their natural family.' We found lots of situations to try and justify our decision, but we always felt that [lack of information] was a difficult issue and still do.

The other thing that we found a bit scary was the idea of having a child who could be very different from us in some way. That can happen anyway but this whole process throws a different light on it. We thought very deeply about what kind of parents we were going to make and it was a real issue for us to be the best parents we possibly could to help our children grow up well adjusted with this little extra factor that's thrown in.

I feel that, apart from counseling, prospective parents should wherever possible seek out parents of donor-conceived children and adults born of donor conception to find out first hand what may lie ahead for them.

Before parents make the final decision to use donor gametes there are many issues they need to look at, such as:

- Have we grieved the loss of our own biological child and the fact that no one will carry on our genetic line?

- Have we grieved the loss of the child that we would have had as a couple?

- Is carrying and giving birth to a child so important to us that we would not consider adoption if it was an option?

- Will we choose an anonymous donor, one who can be identified, or will we find our own donor? What issues does our choice bring with it?

- Will we be able to cope with a pregnancy conceived with the gametes of an anonymous person/a friend/relative?

- Will we tell our child how they were conceived? How and when will we do it?

- Do we tell others – when and who?

- What will we do if our child wants to meet his or her donor?

This list is by no means exhaustive but it does contain some of the important issues that really should be thought about and discussed in depth before deciding on donor conception. Today I am meeting more and more people who have a hunger to know what the long-term issues are. They want to know the truth about what may lie ahead for them if they follow the donor conception path. A good many have already realized that there are serious issues to deal with. They seem so well informed and thoughtful compared to the way I was back in the 1980s. I have also met infertile people in recent times who have looked at these issues and decided that donor conception is not for them. Some have moved on to adoption while others have chosen to remain childless. I applaud these people for the bravery of their decision.

The desire to reproduce and be a parent can be very strong, and it is not often that we analyze why we want to have a child at all. For many of us it just seems like a natural part of life. Fertile couples don't often sit down and discuss their reasons for wanting a child, but people who use donated gametes to create their child sometimes feel the need to analyze their reasons for wishing to be a parent. Is it wanting to be loved, wanting a love object, wanting someone to look after and to look after us in our old age, something to further unite us as a couple, or perhaps just to conform?

Tim knew about his infertility prior to meeting his wife, and this meant that talking about parenting was an inevitable part of getting to know each other.

> I think in raising that I was infertile, it was a natural progression to talk about alternatives. We both seemed to be on the same wavelength in talking about DI and other alternatives. I think both of us really saw having kids as very much a fundamental part of getting married.

In a partnership, things are not always on a totally equal basis and this can also be true of the desire to parent. One person can have a deeper desire to have a child than the other. It is unthinkable for some men to deny their wife the experience of pregnancy and birth, and for this very reason they will sometimes agree to going through with donor conception. Bob had also discovered his infertility some time before he met Glenda.

> I'd actually gotten over the problem of not being able to have children and really didn't consider children an important part of the rest of my life. However, a woman's need for a family or a baby is something men can't understand, and with that in mind I had a 100 percent intention of supporting Glenda through raising a family.

I've often wondered whether my desire to have children was not heightened by the fact that Patrice had two children from his previous marriage. He would always have lifelong ties to his first wife; would my having children put me on a more equal footing? Kara also married a man who had children by his first wife.

> My husband had a vasectomy 16 years ago, a reversal ten years ago, varicocele surgery shortly thereafter. We had three to four inseminations with my husband's sperm before moving on to two IVF attempts, and then deciding that we must now make a decision to give up on having my husband's child. It was more painful to know that I would never have with him what he had with his ex-wife. She had his children and I would never know what our offspring would be like. But he convinced me that it wasn't important, that the child would be ours and that he would love them the same. A part of me wanted so much to believe and a part of me thought he was saying what he thought I wanted to hear.

Donor conception is for most a last resort – we need to be honest about that. It is not a parent's first choice of how to conceive their child. The first choice has been taken away from them. Once this first choice has gone, prospective parents need to take some time to accept the idea of using the gametes of another person and to think about all the issues.

When John and Kate discovered that John was infertile, Kate wasn't sure that using donor sperm was right for them. She worried about one of them being biologically related to the child and the other not. For quite a long time John and Kate thought that the problem lay with John's sperm but eventually they found out that Kate also had serious fertility problems.

I couldn't believe it; I thought how could life be so difficult as to deal so many bad cards in our direction. Then I thought, really this was meant to be, because I was never 100 percent comfortable with using just donor sperm. Before knowing that there was anything wrong with my eggs I had said that I would prefer to use donor embryo or even adoption. Although I had accepted using donor sperm there was always a niggling thought at the back of my mind. I wanted a baby on equal terms. It was a concern to me that a situation might arise in the future when John might feel that he somehow had less of a say in the upbringing of the child. Needless to say, this feeling was totally unfounded. Nevertheless, the decision to use donor embryo was a relief to me. I felt that once more we were on an equal footing.

Julian and Janet also considered the problem of the inequality of biological relationships within the family.

I was willing to think seriously about it but not until we had exhausted our other possibilities, a miracle cure or something. But I think I knew that we would end up using DI eventually. Julian was fairly accepting but he needed more time to come to terms with it. For me, having a child that was biologically mine was really important and for that reason I couldn't really accept the idea of adoption.

Julian's parents were quite strongly opposed to our using donor sperm, partly for religious reasons and also that they felt it was terribly unfair to use DI. They felt that it would be fairer to adopt and have a child that didn't have either of our genetic qualities. That made it harder for Julian, and being Catholic, feeling that you were doing something against the Church's teachings was hard to come to terms with.

There are others who think that donor conception does have advantages over adoption – like Warren, who felt that even though only one parent would be related to the child it was preferable to adopting.

I thought well, if I can't be the genetic father of the kids the only options are adoption and using DI. I thought that if we used DI the kids would at least carry Leonie's genes. It would mean that there would be a link there, a known factor, whereas [in those days] if you adopted kids you wouldn't usually be aware of their genetic background at all. When anyone has kids it's a bit of a lucky dip but it's a bit less of an unknown quantity when you know the background of one of the people who are the genetic parents.

June only wanted to use donated eggs as a last resort, but she and her husband also seriously considered childlessness as an option.

> I'd thought that using donor eggs was a last resort but I didn't think I'd need to do it. I talked to my sister, she's older, and my girlfriend, and when I said, 'Well, I don't seem to have any eggs,' my girlfriend had said to me, 'I'd always be happy to donate eggs.' I thought that's great but I'm sure that something will happen, because I'd managed to fall pregnant before. For the next year I took time out, tried various alternative things. We also thought about what would life be like if we didn't have kids. We went and did some couples courses for ourselves. For us it was a process that brought us closer together. In fact we ended up buying a certain type of house on the basis of probably not having kids.

Nicky and her husband, Holger, did take some time to consider what they were doing and made choices based on their decisions.

> When my husband was given the shock diagnosis of azospermia he immediately asked, 'What about a sperm donor?' It seemed the logical next step for him. We were living in Germany at the time and the doctor's response was, 'You can't do that,' and that was to be a pretty typical response from the medical profession. At first I felt that it was our best solution, as then no one would know, we could have a normal pregnancy. Looking back I know that was a very naive attitude, but when you so desperately want that baby you don't really think about the future consequences.
>
> One doctor did offer to refer us immediately for DI and was surprised at our hesitation. Deep down we must have had reservations and realized that it wasn't the 'quick fix' solution that it appeared to be. We just weren't ready yet. We were still grieving too much.
>
> Gradually, as we made contact with the DCSG, we realized DI was in fact a much more complicated process, and it became very quickly apparent that the child has a right to know [about his or her conception]. The thought of all these future complications made me doubt whether DI was right for us. I just wanted that 'normal' family and that 'normal' future. I got more confused and more depressed. When I honestly thought about it, I didn't like the idea of the DI treatment – an unknown man's sperm inside me, creating a baby with a stranger. I just didn't like

the whole idea. Plus all the negativity in Germany put DI in the realm of only just legal and not very ethical. We felt a bit like freaks for considering it.

Holger was always quite positive and unfazed about fathering a child that was not his biological child. Being in a previous relationship with a woman and her small child had helped this way of thinking. Realistically he knew, and I slowly recognized, that in our case there was DI, adoption, or no children. We knew adoption was a long road and at least with DI we could experience the pregnancy together and give our baby the best possible pre-natal care.

I think the final decision, that DI was OK and we were prepared to deal with it and the future consequences, came when we returned to Sydney and met DCSG members. They were normal people with normal families. We met a grandpa who just doted on his non-biological grandkids – genetics are not all-important. After this we knew DI was OK for us. It is not to say that the pain has gone. I don't think it ever will.

We weren't prepared to try DI in Germany because the doctor chooses the donor for you based on physical characteristics. All you find out is what he is studying [they are all students paid for their services]. Donor anonymity is of the utmost importance and you are encouraged not to tell anyone, especially not the child. Couples I met [in Germany] who had used DI were very fearful, stressed, and amazed when I spoke of the openness most of us believe in in Australia. We were involved in the founding of the first DI support group in Germany, and I hope it will give the support we find here from our group.

We are lucky that we moved [back to Australia] to Victoria to start on the DI program and fall pregnant. At least in this state we have the legislation that at eighteen our child will have access to identifying information about the donor. We've now got two months to go [till the birth]. We've got no regrets about using DI. I know there's a lot ahead of us. We fully believe in honesty, and plan to tell our children the truth and hopefully one day meet the donor. My advice to you is – take your time, DI is not for everyone, and you really have to be ready for it before you start.

Mary and her husband looked way beyond pregnancy and birth before going ahead with DI.

I said several times to Nicholas, 'It's quite OK for you to feel sad about what we're doing.' I wanted to talk to him about the potential children we couldn't have because I didn't want him to think that I was rushing into something just because I wanted to have a baby. We knew that it was a serious thing to undertake. From the point of view of the child it was really important for us to realize that we were making decisions that involved someone else who wasn't there to say whether or not they liked the idea of the decisions we were making. It was a dilemma. We thought, 'What if the child hates us for what we've done?' But in the end we felt that it was OK because we were going to be totally open about it and if the child wanted to know who the donor was we'd make every effort to find out. We also chose a donor who had said he would be happy to meet any offspring later. That was an important consideration for us. We didn't want someone who would want to remain anonymous.

Ralf and his wife decided to go ahead and try DI. He thought about DI from a parenting point of view.

I think DI is not a problem for me. If I met a divorced woman with a child I think I could love her child like my own. With DI we would have a real pregnancy together and also half of the genes would be from us. And who is the father? The biological or the social father? I think the father is the man the child says 'father' to, and that would be me.

The decision to use donor conception may come after many years and attempts with other reproductive technologies such as IVF. Geoff describes the impact the suggestion of using donor conception had on his wife.

The day we found out that we would have to use donor egg to have a baby was terrible. It was fine by me how we had the baby, it didn't matter. I just knew how much my wife had wanted to have a baby, that's all she'd been thinking about for years through all the IVF. I thought she'd be OK with it, but after the doctor told us I looked at her and she had this strange look on her face. She told the doctor she'd have to think about it.

She didn't talk about it all the way home and shut herself in the bedroom when we got home. I could hear her crying and didn't know what to do, what to say to make her feel better. I've never felt that helpless before.

When we finally did sit down and talk about it I told her that we didn't have to have children, that we'd be fine. She kept saying that she wanted to have a baby but the idea of using another woman's eggs scared her. At the same time she also talked so practically about it, she would be able to have the baby grow inside her, she would be able to give birth; the baby would be ours. It was logical, but to her something didn't seem right. She's an only child so this would mean the end of her biological line; she worried not just for herself but how her parents would feel about it.

Mary and Nicholas also looked at donor conception from the point of view of carrying on their genetics.

> When we found out that Nicholas had no sperm we looked at the options that were available to us. We didn't want to adopt, not only because of our age being against us but because we wanted to have a child that we would be related to. We're cousins so if I had a child that was half mine, genetically Nicholas would also be related to it. It would have an eighth of his genes, in theory, and so we both liked that idea. We thought that if donor insemination didn't work we might well consider not having children.

Just because a woman is not in a relationship doesn't mean that her biological urge to have children disappears, but it can mean a lot of serious thought has to go into the decision to 'go it alone.'

> I have to be honest, I have felt depressed a couple of times when I think, 'Why do I have to conceive like this, why can't I just have sex?' I really had to think it through before I proceeded. Children are not toys and they're not accessories. (Debra)

> The thought of not having my own child was frightening. I had always thought of myself as a mother some day, and at thirty-eight, the time had come. I had been in a relationship which ended, and I didn't want to go through that again to find that I still may not have a child. Someone I was talking to happened to mention that you don't have to have a partner to have a child; you could go through a clinic, and that stuck in my mind. I thought about it quite a lot because it is a big responsibility bringing up a child on your own. It was something I didn't want to miss out on even though I knew it was going to be hard and the way I was going to do it was going to be difficult. It wasn't enough to turn me off doing it. It was something I really wanted to do. My GP had asked me what would I do if my parents weren't behind me and I said I didn't think it would stop me doing it, but using hindsight now I think it would have been very hard to do it without them. (Glenda)

Some, like Karen, started thinking about using donor conception from quite an early age.

I decided in my early twenties not to miss out on motherhood if I did not find 'the right one,' so to speak. As I neared thirty and was single (by choice) I looked into DI because I began to feel the pangs of my biological clock. I had always had difficult menstruation with extreme cramps, etc., and was concerned that if I waited too long I might never have children, a thought that was worse than being single for the remainder of my life.

What about a woman who is in a relationship with another woman? Is the decision-making process any different than for a heterosexual couple?

I'd been with my partner for exactly four years when we started talking about children. I know it was exactly four years because it was our anniversary. She brought it up as a single friend of hers had just had a child through donor insemination and we do know other lesbian couples who have had children, one couple that we see regularly have a son who is nearly eight. While the thought of having children had occurred to me I'd always pushed it to the back of my mind. My main concern was what all the relatives would say – it's taken them long enough to accept me and my partner being together. But I know we would make great parents and after talking for a while we thought we should investigate further.

We made an appointment at a clinic about twenty minutes drive away where friends of ours went. The doctor didn't see any problems and sent us to see a counselor. The counselor brought up a lot of things, such as male rolemodels, decision making within the family, how we would answer questions about the child not having a father (we will talk about the love we have for each other) and how we will deal with questions our child might be asked at school. We asked the counselor if she knew of any problems with two women having a child by DI. She said that no one had really done any research that she knew of in this area, but she said that lesbian couples didn't seem to have any more problems with raising children that hetero couples. So we have decided to go ahead. It's scary but it's also exciting. (Jane)

As I have mentioned before, there are heterosexual couples who end up making the decision to remain childless because they are not comfortable with donor conception as a method of creating their family; the same can apply to lesbian couples.

Not long after we met we did talk about having kids some day. It seemed like a great idea. Why shouldn't we, lots of other lesbian couples we knew had done it. We decided we'd wait until we were settled. We ended up buying a house in a lovely neighbourhood with a great local school.

One day we sat down and started talking about having a child. Suzee came from a home with a great mom and dad, she's got a really close relationship with her dad. My parents were divorced when I was twelve. I see my dad (my mom died a few years ago) but we're not especially close. Suzee and I talked about what it would be like growing up not having a dad. We thought maybe we could find a male friend who could donate, but when we looked at all the choices for various reasons none of them seemed right. The idea of using an anonymous donor was almost immediately ruled out, it just didn't seem right. So here we are, we have decided that for us there will be no children, we are a couple and that's it. (Carol and Suzee)

The reasons for choosing to use donor conception are not always because of infertility, or being single, or in a same-sex relationship. There are people who use donated gametes to prevent the passing on of a genetic condition to any children they might have.

John has been living with a genetic condition all his life, a condition that has caused great pain and meant that there were many restrictions in his life. When it came time to think about having children, John had to make a very serious and personal decision.

I have a condition called Epidermolysis Bullosa that in theory is not life threatening – however can be life shortening. I had a biopsy and they said that I had a fifty/fifty chance of passing the condition along. There was no guarantee that it wouldn't skip a generation and that scared me as much as anything as well. My mother had the condition and my sister. My mother's two younger brothers do not have it, and the only reason I'm around is that my sister is older and the doctors said it wouldn't happen to a male. That was back in 1962 when they knew less than the little they know now. Unfortunately, I proved them wrong.

The issue was not about me but what would happen to Emily or Matthew, I can put names to them now but then we couldn't. What would it be like for them? As an adult you can learn to cope with just about anything but as a child it's different. The catalyst for me was when I approached my mother and asked her, 'What do you reckon, should I have a child?' and she said, 'No, do not have a child and risk passing it on.' I asked her, if she could have her time again would she have had me? She replied, 'No, you wouldn't be here.' She said it was just terrible watching a child fall over and just lose skin, and blister, and not be able to play football or go swimming, and not be able to do anything a 'normal' child could. The stares of adults and the taunts of other children were almost as bad.

I can now see where Mum was coming from when I watch the kids and see what they are doing and that they're not hurting themselves from simple bumps. I think, from my own perspective, if I'd put them in that position and they had my condition and were going through all the pain I went through as a child (which I really don't remember that much about) and were scarred for life, I couldn't handle that. I'd rather try and handle any type of rejection that might come later [because of using DI] with them not understanding or rejecting me as a father. I'd rather try and cope with that than put them through the condition that I have all for the sake of it being my sperm and it being my biological child and satisfying my ego. There was a viable alternative there which had less risk; we would just run the normal risk of a healthy or an unhealthy child.

4

Choosing a Donor

> I remember thinking it was like shopping through a mail order catalogue; you can see bits of things but you can never see the whole thing. (Caroline)

Choosing the person who will be the biological parent of your child from a list? It's a pretty strange notion. For most people the person who contributes the egg or sperm to create their child is the person they fell in love with, the person they chat to over breakfast. It's the person whose face is almost as familiar as their own. But for those who are in an infertile relationship or who have no partner the situation is very different.

When they've decided that donor conception is where they are heading a single person or couple then have to make the decision of who their donor will be. Will they get a friend or relative to donate their reproductive material? Will they choose an anonymous donor? Or will they choose a path somewhere in between?

Once upon a time, if a person joined a fertility program there was no choice at all in which donor was used. They got an anonymous donor of the clinic's choosing as Jenny, Glenda, and Anne describe.

> The doctor took physical details of Tom and told us the donor would be chosen accordingly. There was never mention of the donor being someone we knew and it relieved me greatly to be told the donor details would be destroyed in ten years. I look back and see we were a couple wanting a family, but we were not thinking of babies who become children and adolescents with their own rights and questions. Though we got physical details of the donor when Kylie was fifteen and Glenn eleven, I would like the donor's names so they could have them later on, if they wish. (Jenny)

They took down the particulars of Bob and said they would match the donor to him. It was all anonymous. We had to sign a form to say we wouldn't try and find any information about the donor. I was quite happy with that at the time. (Glenda)

We hoped she would be a normal, healthy baby. I had some worries because I didn't know exactly what had been put inside my body and where it had come from. I think that infertile couples should be the ones to choose their own donated sperm and if possible inseminate themselves. It's about regaining control in a situation where you've lost so much control. (Anne)

Catherine conceived more recently but also had no choice of donor.

We gave in some information about our physical characteristics. The hospital then chose the donor and gave us non-identifying information at [the time of] insemination. It was a strange feeling being given this information minutes before the [insemination], almost like an introduction. We know he was a graduate in economics with a great interest in sport and literature. That, plus physical characteristics, is all we are likely to ever know.

How did the use of anonymous donors begin? Before egg or embryo donation existed the idea was that no one needed to know that a man was infertile. A donor was chosen who had physical characteristics similar to the husband. Blood groups were also matched wherever possible to further strengthen the match. If all this was done then perhaps no one, not even the child, would suspect that things were not as they seemed.

Some doctors even went so far as to mix the husband's ejaculate with the donor's so that the couple could hold on to the thought that perhaps the husband had been able to produce that one sperm which fertilized the egg. It was also suggested to couples that they go home immediately after the insemination had been performed and have sexual intercourse. Doctors would tell patients, 'Oh, well, you never know, it might happen.' In Australia I last heard of this happening when told by a couple who went through DI in the late 1980s and had been told by their doctor to go home directly after insemination and make love. In a few places such as the UK and the State of Victoria that have reproductive technology legislation, the mixing of sperm has been forbidden. But I am appalled when I read bulletin board messages on the Internet that mention this practice is still going on in some countries. There appears to be so little thought of what the long-term consequences of doing this might be to all concerned.

On finding that she had conceived with donor sperm mixed with her husband's, one of Cathy's first thoughts was, 'So now I'm pregnant, but with whose sperm?' Cathy's story is further told in Chapter 7 *Treatment, Pregnancy and Birth.*

Not having a choice of donor was all part of the secrecy and anonymity that once totally surrounded donor conception. Claudia and Ralf live in Germany and visited a number of doctors in their attempts to conceive a child by donor insemination. Claudia talks about the secrecy of DI.

> First, we thought about adoption. The woman in the youth welfare department was so unfriendly on the phone that we didn't go further. I asked my gynecologist for other possibilities and she gave us the address of a doctor, 40 kilometres away, who did DI. We had six attempts but they all failed. The problem was that we had only one day to come to him. I was so excited that my ovulation was no longer regular. We paid 400DM for every attempt. He told us nothing about the donors. He only told us that they were in good health. He warned us not to talk about it. He said, 'If you have your baby in your arms, you will forget where it is from.'
>
> At this time it was our secret, we didn't tell anybody except one person (my best friend). Then the doctor retired, and his successor did no DI.
>
> We got another address for a doctor here in Stuttgart. When we met him it was the first and the last time. He proposed that we ask Ralf's father to give his sperm so that it would be in the family and much cheaper. He said that Ralf's father would die eventually and so the problem would be solved (no one would ever have to know we used someone else's sperm). It was horrible.

While donation of sperm and eggs is not uncommon within families it is usually from a brother, sister or cousin. The idea of inter-generational donation is frowned upon by many counselors. The worry can be that in extreme cases it carries the hint of incest and at the very least can upset family generational balances. In the case of Claudia and Ralf, if they had used Ralf's father's sperm their child would also have been Ralf's brother.

In the last ten years or so people like myself have been allowed some choice in donors. At the first clinic we attended Patrice and I were given about half-a-dozen cards which had brief physical descriptions of men who had given their sperm. The description outlined their eye, skin and hair colour, weight range, and blood group, that was it. There wasn't one which was an exact match to Patrice so in the end it almost became a case of 'eeny, meeny, miny, mo.' I felt very strange, as though I was doing something slightly improper.

Barbara and Paul found it very hard to make a decision as well.

> We were given about three or four donors to choose from with very limited information about each. It was virtually impossible to choose, because you wanted a blueprint of your husband and that's not available. They're such unemotive issues: hair colour, eye colour, etc. You want to know more, such as does he like football, or does he fly a kite? It's virtually impossible because when it's down to comparing the same features, like the height or the eye colour, they all sound the same anyway; you just think basically, 'Who cares, just give me one of them.'

It's quite normal to expect that once we choose a donor to match our husband that the child will resemble our husband in some way. It doesn't always work out that way. Our children were conceived by three different donors all chosen to match my husband. I expected to have three children with dark hair. Our daughter is blonde and both sons were born blond, one has since darkened to mid-brown.

Barbara and Paul were given a donor who did not match Paul that well and they expected that their child would turn out to match the donor's description.

> Jake doesn't resemble the description of the donor, he's more like me when I was little, he's got the same colour hair and he's flat strap [very thin] like I was and he's about the same build as I was. Jake's got blond hair and blue eyes, Barbara has blue eyes and I had blond hair when I was little. His hair is starting to darken up a bit like mine. (Paul)

In the last few years many clinics have been giving prospective parents who are making their choices a great deal more information on the donors. Now recipients often get information about education, sports, hobbies, religious and ethnic backgrounds, and sometimes the donor has also written something about his reasons for donating. This has come about for many reasons: pressure from prospective parents to have some control over a situation that has left them feeling helpless and very much out of control, and a growing awareness on the part of prospective parents that when they tell their children about their conception they will need information with which to answer their children's questions. Parents want to use a donor about whom they have some information beyond basic physical characteristics.

While having this extra information may help in the future it does not necessarily make the choice easier, as Vivianne describes.

> It was funny, they all seemed quite intelligent, one was a lawyer, one was an electronic engineer, and the other was a father of four children, but he was red haired and I thought no, there's no red hair in our family. We want our kids to fit in so they can choose who they want to tell, so they're not being bombarded with questions because they look different. Then there was the choice between the lawyer and the single guy. I said to Michael either one would be good. I went for the sporting one; he was into scuba diving, gym instructing – if he's really fit he would pass on healthy genes.

Single women who use anonymous sperm to create their families have no one to match a donor to. What criteria do they use when selecting a donor? Glenda, Lois and Deborah describe how they chose their donors.

> I selected similar characteristics to me in eye colour and height because I'm quite tall. I don't know whether pastimes and interests are inherited or something that just happens but I'm not very sporty so I looked for someone who wasn't overly sporting but had some sort of sport interest as well as cultural. It was the strangest experience, having a selection of donors in front of me and saying, 'Oh, I like that one.' It's not the sort of experience you should be laughing about but I just found it amusing that I was sitting here with a list of sperm donors and their characteristics and choosing one to have a child by. (Glenda)

> I went to a private clinic that had their own donors as well as flying in donated sperm from other regions in Canada. I described the appearance and background of men that I usually dated and was told that they had donors who were matches, or close matches, to my description. They told me of the donor's height, weight, hair and eye colour, educational back-

ground and heritage. I chose a gentleman that had already been success-ful (my second donor – my first was flown in and was not working) since this was my ninth attempt and I wanted to be sure to get sperm 'worth the money,' so to speak! I also chose this man because he was an engineer, as were my father and brother (and I am more on the artistic and dreamy side). I hoped he would create a nice balance (which seems to be the case). (Lois)

I would have liked more choice; I would have loved an Asian donor. The doctor gave me about fifteen cards. I wiped out most of them on the spot as I looked through them and saw people with cancer in the immediate family. I ended up taking home five or six and they were the ones which looked really solid.

I would have liked more information on the donor I chose because he left the family medical history section blank, but then he was a medical student and if there were any problems he would have written that down. The card had hobbies, sports, interests, height, build, hair colour, eye colour. He was Russian Caucasian, a medical student, which is a big plus because I'm not good at science. I chose someone with a science back-ground because I have the business and creative skills but am useless at science. I know he likes reading and is a little bit creative, so I know he's not boring or stick in the mud. When I looked at the cards I wanted someone with a medium build who was a bit taller than me. He has a light build and is five foot ten. The nurse at the clinic said to me, 'He's young, he's in his twenties, he's got a light frame, it'll spread, he'll turn into a medium.' He met the rest of my criteria. Out of all the cards they gave me there was no one else who filled the criteria as neatly.

This guy I've chosen has been on the program for a while, apparently he makes the world's most beautiful babies and that actually put me off. I thought for the first time, 'Oh, my God, there's going to be little half-brothers and half-sisters that we'll never know, how strange.' They limit how many people can use each donor, which gives some meagre form of reassurance. (Deborah)

There is a move in a number of countries to increasingly use donors who are already known to the recipient parents or who are willing to be identi-fied in future. An identifiable donor is the middle ground between using an anonymous donor and a known donor. This type of donor will be anony-mous to the parents at the time of conception but has agreed to be identi-fied to the child when he or she reaches adulthood. The state of Victoria has legislated to ensure that only this type of donor is used at clinics within that state. (There are three other states of Australia who appear to be also moving towards using only identifiable donors.) It is also the only type of donor used in Sweden and New Zealand.

It is not unusual nowadays to find people who select a clinic because it only uses identifiable donors. Some parents feel that the choice of knowing the donor is then the child's and not the parents'. Christina and her partner decided that using an identifiable donor was an option for them.

> My partner and I have both wanted children ever since we got together (approximately eight years ago), but we decided to feel really settled before we pursued the whole thing. My partner was a little worried about using a known donor in the beginning but has since decided that it will be the best for the child. We attended a 12 week parenting class together, we know other lesbian women and their older children and have had many discussions about what is really important to us, and then in turn to the child, who we believe in our circumstance has the right to know. I am saying 'our circumstance' because we are lesbians and have known a few other children who have expressed the importance of knowing their biological father. So with this (as well as my own feelings on things, especially my intuition which tells me our particular child will want to know) we decided to pursue the idea of having a known donor.
>
> We looked at many options and were going to use a sperm bank that is available in California, where after the child is between 3–12 months old you are able to contact the bank and then in turn are able to have contact with the donor. This was an option that we were seriously considering, until we came across a guy who was advertising on the web, on a donor site…which was a little weird at first for my partner and me. We have been speaking to him for about a year now and know lots about him. So, we are going to go ahead and use him to inseminate. We are really excited because we are going to meet him in person in the near future, with further contact to be discussed.

After having one child by donor conception parents have to decide if they should stop there, is their family complete? If the answer is no then they have to find out if they can use the same donor again.

When we were conceiving our first child Patrice and I thought that it would probably be our only child, but later, when we decided to enlarge our family, we switched to another clinic which was closer to home and the opportunity to use the same donor was not available. At the time, using a different donor did not appear to be a problem and no one at the clinic suggested otherwise. We were not to realize for many years what implications this could have for our children.

Ken and Rose thought ahead and wanted to use the same donor for subsequent siblings.

> Ken and I chose the donor and then Ken went overseas on business. We had a couple of goes with the chosen donor but then one day the nurse said, 'If this treatment doesn't work, that's the end of the straws from that donor.' I said, 'What?' One of the things we had discussed was that we hoped we would have two children from the same donor. This was obviously not to be, so without Ken's company I had to choose another donor. I made sure there were lots of straws because they seemed to dish them out to multiple recipients, and without warning they would be gone.
>
> We had a few treatments with the new donor and I fell pregnant with our first child. Before the baby was born we paid $400 and signed a contract to have thirty or so straws put away for us. About three months after the birth I rang up the clinic and said, 'I'm getting on in age so we would like to wean this child and try for another.' A week later I got a letter in the post saying that due to an administrative error it was regretted that there were no longer any straws available from our donor. They had been lost.
>
> Ken and I went in to see the clinic director. To his credit, he viewed the situation very seriously. He tracked down every straw from that donor and who had received them; he was very thorough. He rang us back and said he'd found 13 straws from our donor, inadvertently stored in the hepatitis B tank. We said that it didn't sound all that great being stored in the hep. B tank. He said that if he and his wife were in the same situation they would use the straws. He said any danger of contamination was very, very small. Of course we just have to believe that those straws were our original ones inadvertently stored. Maybe one day we'll have our boys genetic relationship checked.

Leonie and Warren had no choice in the donors of their first two children but when they decided to have a third child there was a decision to make.

Geraldine's donor was chosen for us, we got no information on him and we accepted that, which we feel a little sad about, but in those days we didn't question things at the clinic. We also didn't choose the donor of our second child but we received non-identifying information later when we asked for it. For our third child we could have used the same donor but his AIDS test came back inconclusive twice. We decided that we would use another different donor because we also thought, 'How would Geraldine feel if the other two are full siblings?' Once again we had no information apart from hair colour, etc. and we had to ask for a bit more non-identifying information later.

The idea of using a known donor such as a relative or friend as opposed to an anonymous donor is a worry for some. Will the donor interfere in their lives? Will the child be confused about who his parents are? Will the child reject a parent in favour of the donor?

Many people who contemplate using a known donor first think about a relative, as Julian describes.

After I came to terms with infertility, the first thing I thought was, 'We'll get a cousin from Italy to donate sperm, it will be perfect because we'll keep the genetics of the family.' Initially we thought it was a fantastic idea because my cousins are on the other side of the world, they shouldn't mind, we'll just send them a letter and ask them if they could donate.

But when we thought of the actual idea of sending a letter to a cousin that I'd never met and asking him for something like sperm we couldn't do it. It took a long time to get used to the idea of an anonymous donor, but then I saw some advantages in having somebody outside the family completely. If we used a cousin and then later on they couldn't have kids of their own there could be complications.

Using a relative or friend to be a donor brings some obvious advantages: genetic links (when using a relative of the infertile person), not having to worry about what the donor is like, control (the parents choose their own donor, not the clinic) and perhaps most importantly of all the child will have the opportunity to know their donor and have any questions answered. The idea of a child having a family biological link is very important to many people, but just because we would like to use a family member doesn't always make it possible.

Ken has three brothers; he rang each of them to propose that they consider being our donor. They each confirmed that they would help. We'd not considered whether to select one or all, or indeed even if they were able to be a donor. Ken said to his brothers, 'This isn't like putting the concrete down on Saturday, this is something which is going to affect us for the rest of our lives so take a period of time to think about it.' One brother's wife said it was not to be discussed again. Another brother's wife had had a hysterectomy and couldn't bear that we would have children who were her husband's and she couldn't. The other brother had a partner who supported him in helping us and he did have a sperm test in preparation. The sperm count was very low. (Rose)

Some people feel that a friend may make a suitable donor.

I had been through my third IVF attempt when the clinic found that my husband had absolutely no sperm. It hit us both like a ton of bricks. We had good friends near the clinic and after treatments we would call in there and cry on their shoulders. My girlfriend's a nurse and she understood what was happening. When I rang her to tell her what had happened we joked about her husband's features being exactly the same as my husband's. Personality wise, they are totally different but in looks very similar. We made a joke about her husband working only a few blocks away from the clinic; if only he could whip round here in his lunchtime we'd be right. Next thing you know she said, 'That's not such a silly idea.' She talked to her husband when he came home from work and he said yes.

We actually started some inseminations ourselves but it wasn't successful and after a while our friends decided they couldn't continue. I was a little disappointed but they were still good friends and we just appreciated what they had done for us, they kept our spirits up. I'm pretty embarrassed now but we didn't think through the implications, we didn't really know what we were doing. We didn't discuss what would happen after the baby was born. Maybe I thought it would frighten them away.

Perhaps one of the main obstacles to using known donors is not knowing what the etiquette is. How do you ask someone to be your donor or do you wait for them to offer? If you find someone, how do you behave towards them before and after the birth? There are no guidelines for this situation but there are some parents who have found their way through this largely unexplored area and created their families using a known donor. Lynette describes why and how she and her husband came to use a friend as a sperm donor.

Because of our professional background with children in care, we believed it was imperative that any child we had was able to identify their parents, both parents, and so artificial insemination by unknown donor was not an alternative we wanted to consider.

We considered our options – there was no near male relative on my husband's side of the family whom we could approach. Fortunately, though, we have a wonderfully close friend who, coincidentally, looks very much like my husband. They are often mistaken for brothers. He is intelligent, gentle, kind and funny, with lots of other positive qualities. After some deliberation we decided that if we couldn't have a child that was biologically linked to my husband, then having one who was biologically linked to someone we both loved and respected would be our next preferred option.

We were concerned about what his response would be to our request, and how this arrangement might impact upon our friendship. He had a new woman in his life – what would she make of this odd request? We explained to him our predicament and why we wanted his help; what it would mean to a child to have such a special person as his biological father; and what it might mean for him. We left him to think about it for a while and to talk it over with his girlfriend. Needless to say, we were thrilled and relieved when they both came back to us saying they would be delighted to assist.

At first, being the stubbornly independent people that we are, and having a wonderfully co-operative doctor, we decided to try self-insemination. And surprisingly we had success relatively quickly. Unfortunately that first pregnancy was ectopic, leaving me very ill and requiring the removal of one tube. After many more frustrating months I discovered that my remaining tube was blocked and our only hope was going to be IVF.

Our next challenge was to convince the ethics committee of the clinic that we should be permitted to use a known donor. It was not common practice at that time (although we were aware of at least one clinic that was doing it), and despite our well-reasoned argument citing all the appropriate research, the ethics committee refused our request. We felt so strongly about the right of our offspring to have access to their origins (which the clinics would not guarantee) that we decided to fight. We had discovered that the same clinic which denied our request was allowing known egg donors, but not known sperm donors. That was hypocritical and discriminatory, so we threatened them with legal action under the anti-discrimination legislation and appealed to the Minister for Health to intervene. Finally, but not graciously, they relented and acceded to our request. We now have two healthy, well-adjusted children. They have a wonderful relationship with their 'special uncle', his wife and their son, and they know why he is special, and how they came into being. Our son looks a bit like his 'special uncle', especially when he pulls a particular face, but then he looks a lot like his dad as well.

Deborah and her husband approached a relative and asked him to donate.

My husband and I are starting the process of DI with a known donor, his brother. My husband has a rare genetic disease (that his brother was spared) that causes brain tumors. We have decided not to pass this lovely disease on, so even before we were married his brother agreed to be the donor.

Approaching my brother-in-law during a visit, my husband talked to him briefly and then the four of us (his wife too) sat down and talked. They asked why we chose him (as opposed to my husband's other two brothers). After some joking about his good looks, we explained that it was because he didn't have kids and wasn't planning to have them, so it was less weird with having half-siblings, etc. We did a lot of the talking and they said they'd think about it.

We called them later and his brother said, 'Sign me up.' They said they would be aunt and uncle, though they admit that this child will be special to them. They are happy to answer any questions the child has and hope to have a close and loving relationship with him or her.

There is very little anonymous egg donation as compared with anonymous sperm donation. That is not to say that anonymous egg donation doesn't go on. In some countries large amounts of money can change hands for eggs, and in some clinics IVF patients can be encouraged to 'share' their eggs in return for reduced fees or to move up a waiting list.

The vast majority of egg donors in Australia are either friends or relatives of the person they are donating to. Even those women who donate to someone they don't know often feel that it is important to either meet the recipients before donation or are willing to share information on a long-term basis. June describes how she and her husband, Graeme, became parents through egg donation.

We decided to use my sister as an egg donor. She went through the tracking and I was having injections to get my body ready. They thought the best chance would be to use a fresh embryo. My body did respond, but hers didn't. They thought they would only get one, maybe two, eggs but when she went in for an egg pick-up they couldn't find any. That was really quite devastating for both me and my sister. It was very much a shared thing.

After that process my girlfriend again offered to be an egg donor but at that stage I felt that it had to be a family member. It was partly to do with my genetics and partly to do with my family continuing on. So again we stepped back from the process and discussed the other option, which was using a donor embryo, but I felt that I was choosing to have a baby with my husband, and if it couldn't be half my genetic material then I wanted it to be half his.

At that point I decided that if I was going to use donor eggs and they couldn't be my sister, then I would rather that they were from someone I didn't know. We decided that we would advertise for a donor egg. We talked to the clinic about it and they decided that they would help us and we came up with an ad. At that time my girlfriend and her husband sat me down and my girlfriend said, 'Look, I don't think you're taking us seriously, I've got my family, I've got my two kids, I don't want to have any more. I've talked to my mother about it (her father had passed away). We're all really comfortable with it.' I was like, 'Oh, I don't know at the moment.'

We offered to look after their kids (who were at that stage about four years and eighteen months) to let them have a night off and go and stay in a hotel. Over that weekend I went through this whole change, I was looking after a baby boy and I found myself, on the second day, thinking, 'This is what I want to be doing; this is what having a baby is about. He's my friend's baby but I still love him.'

After that weekend we had our friends over for dinner and sat down and talked about [egg donation], they were really keen, they had given it a huge amount of thought as well. But my friend was still worried about some things, like what would happen when the baby's born and she would want to give me advice because she's my girlfriend and she's already got babies, how would we feel about that? How would I handle that? I was worried about that too. I was worried about when my child gets to be a teenager, and as teenagers do might not want me as their parent, wishes they were adopted and wants to go and live with her. Her view was that she would say to them, 'Well, I love you dearly but actually you wouldn't exist if it wasn't for your mother and father. Yes, I've helped your mum by giving her a cell to have you but you're their child.' And so we talked about lots of things and decided that yes, it was something we'd all like to do.

I went into the clinic and picked up all the information that I could get for donors including issues to think about. We got stuff off the Internet; we got information about all the ins and outs of how we'd feel. We felt that it was a decision that all four of us were making.

In a similar vein Andrew and Bronwyn, after not being able to use their first donor, also had someone come to them with an offer of donation.

We spent three dreadful days contemplating the loss of our first donor when a phone call came out of the blue with another offer. Two friends said that their daughter would like to offer herself as a donor. We were surprised and overwhelmed. I had to choke back tears as I spoke to them.

Her mother explained how they had been watching a film on a surrogate pregnancy. Afterwards, they discussed the film as they washed the dishes. Her daughter said that she couldn't give up a child that she had carried but she wouldn't mind donating her eggs to someone who couldn't conceive herself. Her mother smiled and said that she knew someone who needed an egg donor. She made an offer to us, acting through her parents to take some of the pressure off us while we considered our options. As we were already friends with our new donor, we accepted very quickly. (Andrew)

I feel, now, that there are huge advantages to using a known donor as opposed to an anonymous or identifiable donor. The fear of the unknown would be gone. Our child, and we ourselves, would be able to have a relationship with the donor which would allow the sharing of information. My two eldest children would know the answer to the question they have both asked about their donors: 'What is his name?'

5

Donors

Years ago I used to donate blood and would walk out of the blood bank proudly wearing the sticker given to me which read, 'Be nice to me, I gave blood today.' Imagine if stickers like that were given to sperm and egg donors: 'Be nice to me, I donated sperm today.' Men and women who donate their reproductive tissue are rarely recognized in any public way.

Very few people have knowingly met a sperm or egg donor. We may chat very easily about blood donation and boast about how many donations we've made, but when it comes to the donation of reproductive tissue there is suddenly a reluctance, a certain hesitancy about what can and cannot be asked or discussed. Much of this reluctance can probably be attributed to a lack of knowledge about gamete donation and donor conception.

Sperm Donors

When fresh semen was being used for donor insemination before the mid 1980s it had to be collected very close to the time of insemination and clinics sometimes went to elaborate lengths to keep donors and recipients apart. If the clinic was part of a hospital, then semen was often collected in a separate building, but if this was not possible donors would use a 'back' door.

John donated from the early to mid 1980s in the USA and he describes his experiences of donating fresh semen.

> In those days, doctors scheduled a 'warm' that is, unfrozen donation because the success rate per cycle was 25 percent (compared to 20 percent for frozen sperm). The HIV tests were just coming into use at the end of my donating.

Interestingly, since I was donating 'warm' for a woman probably just down the hall, I could tell if a woman used my sperm two or three cycles in a row, and during some months I knew there were two women separated by a week or two.

One historical tidbit is that I actually produced the sample at my home! The nurse gave me a supply of little bottles. She would call and say simply, 'I need you next Tuesday and Thursday.' I would write her name in my calendar and masturbate into the bottles that morning, attach a label with my 'code,' then drive to the clinic with the jar in my pocket to keep it warm, especially on cold days.

In those days it was considered in the best interests of all parties that they know nothing about each other. Although donor insemination is becoming a more open subject, sperm donors still rarely if ever meet the people who receive their semen. Donors and women awaiting treatment don't sit in the same waiting room. They can only imagine each other because, even today, in most countries the vast majority of sperm donation is still done on an anonymous basis.

In years gone by the most common source of sperm was young medical students. They were convenient, infertility clinics often being at large hospitals and they were known to the doctors. For some students the money paid to them for their donation was easy money, others may have felt that it would be good to help infertile people. For others it may have been subtley suggested by their lecturers as being a worthy thing to do.

Times are changing, there is a growing trend in most countries for donors to be older, married and to already have their own children. This is most marked in countries that have enacted legislation to give rights to donor offspring to access information on their donors.

What is it that makes a man perform the very personal act of masturbation in a clinical setting, an act that will possibly create a new life, a person who will be raised by someone they have never met? Kevin describes what led up to his decision to become a sperm donor.

My wife and I tried to have children for about six years and we couldn't. She had a couple of operations and drug treatment and they ended up working out that she had endometriosis. Finally we put our name down on the IVF waiting list – before we got to the top of the list Robyn got pregnant naturally. We had a couple of children but because we had been on the IVF waiting list we were getting newsletters from the clinic every three months. I noticed in one of the newsletters they were asking for sperm donors. We had a lot of trouble having children and were lucky enough to have a couple. Robyn and I talked about it and decided that I would go and donate. That's how it all came about.

Both Robyn and myself went into the counselor at the hospital where the clinic was and had to fill out a form with minor things on it, like parents, grandparents, occupation, age, colour of hair, eyes and all that sort of thing. It was back in about '86. Things have probably changed quite a bit. I knew that it was anonymous, the counselor talked about the possibility that in years to come they might want people to reveal their identity. That would never be any problem.

Others have been initially attracted by the money but have still thought about helping others.

I was married, the only wage earner in the household and four children to support, money was tight and I saw an ad for a private hospital where they requested donors. They normally target students, but they welcomed me to go along and have a chat. I was thirty-four at the time.

Well, they gave me counseling, discussed future issues that might develop, and asked would I give details for any future offspring in case they sought contact. I saw no problem with that. Then I had to give blood and sperm samples so they could test for disease. The scrape taken from inside my penis was particularly painful! They quizzed me about my health and family history. The counseling made me realize how fortunate I was, as a healthy man, to be able to help others in need.

A few weeks later, they told me that my sperm count was high, so I could begin giving samples. This entailed going into a room with a sample bottle. They provided some girlie magazines to help the process along. I gave samples for two years, and then the limit [of donations] for an individual was reached. (Paul)

Ian had similar reasons to Paul's:

My wife was in hospital, she'd just had the baby or was just about to, and I saw an ad in the paper. We didn't have much money and they were paying $12.00 a donation. I went about it by going into the hospital and asking about it, volunteered and went ahead with it. I didn't have my wife's permission, which was probably a mistake, but I didn't want to bother her with it because she was having a difficult time with the baby. It wasn't necessary at the time to get my wife's permission, and I didn't think she would have any problems with that, because she was a pretty open sort of person too.

Some men find the idea of accepting money for helping infertile people somewhat uncomfortable. I have heard of donors who have refused payment and also a couple who have never cashed cheques given to them by the clinic.

The number of men who already have their own children and are donating sperm appears to be increasing but what of those who do not have children? Why do they donate? Well, probably for similar reasons to men with children but also for another reason. As Greg puts it: 'To help others and become a father as I am not one through marriage or a relationship.'

The need to reproduce one's genes can be very strong, we recognize this in women and talk about a woman's biological clock ticking, but rarely do we think that men too can have an urge to have children. While women in many countries today can use donor insemination through clinics to have children without having a partner, this course of action is naturally not an option for men. John explains how he felt.

> I was a twenty-three year old law student at a top five law school. I had been engaged to be married, but my fiancee broke it off. When my dream of the spouse, kids and house with white picket fence was not coming true, I remembered a classified ad in the student paper seeking donors. I called the clinic mostly as an outlet for a biological imperative I felt. I wanted to reproduce my genes. I thought about it in terms of what we now call evolutionary biology (then sociobiology). I figured, I'm a smart, good-looking, healthy guy and if I were a donor offspring that is the kind of donor I would be grateful for. I was metaphysically involved, too, in wanting a great life for the kids. Caring about them, imagining them running around as children and growing up. Hoping that their parents would be good and loving ones.
>
> Initially they paid me $25 and later $40 cash. I thought it was funny; I would have done it for free. I treated it as 'beer money,' and it was a lot back then.

In the past sperm donors were encouraged to donate and then forget. If a man showed an interest in the future results of his sperm donations he ran the risk of not being accepted as a donor. No counseling was available and very little information was provided.

> They did a full check up on me; they wanted to know about any family medical history, it seemed to be pretty thorough. I didn't speak to a counselor or anyone at the clinic about the long-term issues. I think they just wanted someone to donate; that was their priority. When I first donated I didn't really think about what it all meant, not until I got married and had my own child; once my daughter was born then I thought it might be really nice to meet the other children. (Mike)

> In those days, there was no mention of anything other than anonymity. The doctor assured me, without my asking, that I would not have parental responsibilities. He said there was a legal case in California upholding the donee's husband's obligations.

> I asked about the files, which obviously had my name and medical report. He said they threw them away after a couple years. I said, 'You can't do that.' He shrugged and said, 'Well, we do.' I don't regret the anonymity, but I do wish there had been a mechanism for becoming a 'Yes Donor' at a later date. (John)

A great many clinics now provide counseling for sperm donors to ensure that they are as informed as possible of all the legal and social implications of donation. What rights do donors have? Some clinics are now involving donors by giving them choices such as who their sperm will go to. There are some donors who would like to donate only to heterosexual couples, their thoughts being that they would like the child to grow up with a father and a mother. Donors may also prefer to donate only to a certain religious or ethnic grouping. Also, some would like to limit their donations to one or two families, but the clinics that offer some or all of these choices are not many.

There are men who donate in a known situation; this can be to a couple who are friends or relatives, or to a single woman or lesbian couple. Some people may want to use a donor who also carries the 'family genes.' Michael has donated sperm within his own family. The first insemination was not successful but they will continue to try.

> I donated sperm to my twin brother and his wife. Chris had cancer when he was a kid, he was lucky enough to survive that but he could never have

kids of his own. I felt it a bit strange giving sperm but I've got a son and a daughter of my own and wanted to do something for Chris.

Others just don't want to go down the anonymous path. John talks about the possibility of donating to a single friend.

> I have been in some discussions about becoming a known donor and non-custodial father for a single friend who lives across the country. We have touched on the idea of everything from cryobanking (for six months, with all the doctors and nurses and the expense) to me donating in a jar in the next room, to having sex the old fashioned way, which carries emotional complications for relationship reasons I won't go into.
>
> We are comfortable about the HIV/STD dimension, and are not planning to use a doctor to insulate me from paternity. We will draw up some form of contract to proceed. In fact, I will be non-custodial daddy (custodial if something happens to her) and involved in visiting and paying child support (which I am lucky to be able to afford.) So it will, ideally, be like a post-divorce situation but without the hostile baggage.

Paul is also donating to a single woman with the approval of his wife.

> I currently give samples to an unmarried woman who is forty-three and desperate for a child of her own. The single woman responded to a posting on a DI mailing list I joined. We met, chatted about her situation, and drew up a contract waiving my rights as a father and also stating that she did not intend to make any claim for financial support. As she is a solicitor, she did this herself! I agreed with her that I would not be involved in a future child's life.
>
> She miscarried a year ago and she is trying various fertility avenues, but we meet at regular intervals. She read somewhere that the natural method is the best, so that is what we do. She books a hotel room and we do the necessary there close to or on her ovulation day. It did feel strange at first, but I regard it as strictly an act, there are no feelings involved either way.

A question often asked by parents and donors themselves is how long can a donor donate, how many children can he help to create? There is no definitive answer to this, it very much depends on the clinic and the legislation (if any) of the country. Today those states or countries that have legislation in this area are tending to limit the use of sperm from one donor to five or ten families. In the past there was usually no legal limits on the number of children being born from one donor. While most clinics may have set their own limits there is anecdotal evidence of cases where a donor may have been used to create hundreds of children. Donors have also been known to donate at more than one clinic, as Mike did over a number of years.

> I donated from 1979 to 1984 but it wasn't continuously. When I told a clinic that I had donated before at another clinic they said, 'That's no problem, there's a shortage of donors.'

Whether to tell other people can be a difficult decision for many donors given that it is not an openly discussed subject in our society. Most men choose to keep the information that they have been donors private.

> I don't bring it up unless it comes up in the general conversation. If they're single blokes I might say, 'Have you thought about being a sperm donor?' (Mike)

> I have told my brother and my partners, but not my parents and only a very few friends. (John)

Many clinics now insist that where a man has a wife or partner that they are involved in the decision to donate. If a man has children with his partner then their children will be half-siblings to any the man may have by donation. Even without the encouragement of clinics for partners to be involved in decision making there are sperm donors who have chosen to be open with partners. Greg, who doesn't have a partner, says, 'I would tell a future partner because I try to be open and honest in life.' And others seem to be just as open.

> My wife was happy for me to be a donor, as our financial needs were great at the time I was going to the clinic. (Paul)

Telling a partner does not always go well though. Ian donated while his wife was pregnant and did not discuss it with her at the time.

> I didn't tell her until probably four or five months after the birth [of our daughter]; she didn't react very well actually. When the time came I was surprised she made a sort of mountain out of a molehill. It's all history now; she held it against me, and four or five years after that we divorced.

Of course the reaction could have been very different if the discussion had occurred before the decision to donate was made.

What about other family members. It seems that most donors tend not to tell many other relatives, but Mike was more open than most.

> Yes, they all know about it, I think my mum and dad were a bit stunned because they're Sri Lankan and that sort of thing is just not heard of. They were quite surprised to think that they might have grandchildren that they'll probably never see, it's a bit sad. My wife and daughter, they're quite comfortable with it. My daughter, who's eleven said she would quite love to meet any of her half-brothers or half-sisters, because she's an only child. We think it would be wonderful to meet any of the children if it was ever possible.

The majority of sperm donors I have spoken to over the years have also told their own children about being a donor, as Ian and Kevin describe.

> I told her [nineteen year old daughter] about three years ago now, after I'd seen an article in the newspaper about a young woman who was looking for her donor father. When I told my daughter, my only child, she was really tickled by it, said she'd love to meet her half-siblings if the opportunity came. (Ian)

> I've got four children, the three older ones are fourteen, thirteen, eleven and the young one is only just turned five. I said to my wife that I'd be telling them. I'd been to two or three of these different meetings [of the Donor Conception Support] and they said it's best to tell the kids when they're young. My wife works as a nurse a couple of nights a week and this particular night when she was out I sat them down and said, 'I want to tell you something – first of all do you know about the birds and the bees?' and they're all saying, 'Yeah, yeah.' The young bloke, he was four, he said, 'Oh, yeah, I know all about the birds and the bees, I got stung by a bee last year.' That's what he knew about them. Anyway, I told them that I'd been a sperm donor, that there were 14 offspring and they said nothing. They weren't too interested. All they wanted to do was go back to watching 'Neighbours' on TV.

With the imparting of this type of information to their own children, donors have often been faced with inevitable questions such as: 'How many other children are there?', 'Are they boys or girls?' While most clinics in decades past would not impart to donors information on numbers of offspring, there has been a radical change in recent times. There are now some clinics that automatically let their donors know about any births resulting from their donations. There are also others who will gladly give information when asked. More and more donors are interested in knowing when children are born and what sex they are.

> About three years ago they said four and these were all girls. They gave me the ages, the years they were born, two of them were in one family; that's all they told me. I said I'd be OK to be contacted if any of them wanted to know who their biological father was. (Ian)

Ian's thoughts about being happy to have contact with any offspring are mirrored by many others. Kevin talks about his thoughts.

> The first offspring weren't born till 1990 but what I've done is I've written a letter, maybe five or six pages of information about myself, outlining my physical characteristics, social history, reasons for donating. I've sent a copy of that in to the counselor at the hospital. You're probably looking at 2008 before those children would want information and if any parents want information it's there now, they can just go back to the unit where they had treatment. If any of them [offspring] want to meet that's fine.
>
> I think with so many – 14 children and ten families – I could expect some might want to make contact. That's probably going to be my biggest problem, remembering all the names and parents names. I was a bit bewildered when I found out it was ten families.
>
> I never knew anything for years and years until one day the counselor actually rang me up (this would be in about 95/96) and there had been some pregnancies from the donations. She said they'd run out of sperm and one couple was trying to have another child using the same donor and would I still be able to donate? In that phone call I actually found out that there were some children conceived. Originally, when I donated, we talked about the numbers of children and the counselor asked me how many would I be happy with. I'd never really thought about it. The counselor said, 'We suggest about ten to fifteen' and I said, 'Well, that's fair enough with me.' So the actual number of children born doesn't really worry me. But it represents ten families and if I had my time over again I'd probably ask to donate to five families.

Mike, who donated at more than one clinic, knows he also has a number of children from his donations.

I've been told 15 but I don't know for sure, you get told these things but they don't put anything in writing. I asked one clinic, I said, 'Is it possible for you to tell me how many I've fathered?' They told me that I'd fathered six, three boys and three girls.

John has made a guess at the possible number of children from his fresh semen donations in the 1980s and would be quite happy to make himself known to them.

I asked about the success rate, but was never told about any particular successes. The nurse said that many times people move away or never report back about the birth. Five years later, I went through my old calendars and made a list of the days I donated. Because it was a fresh insemination, I was able calculate approximate birth dates for any successful inseminations (often grouped two days apart for, I presume, one recipient). Statistically there should be five or six children from my donations.

I would be overjoyed and would welcome them with open arms. I began thinking about how to make myself known and accessible about ten years ago. I called around to fertility groups and asked if there was any 'registry', but to no avail. When the Internet emerged, I studied the 'adoptee-birth parent' registries and have thought about setting one up. I also researched DNA paternity matching, which was not available when I donated. I have drafted a form to fill out, with everything one could disclose about the donation to help find matches. One factor in my case is that I do not yet have any children of my own. I would be eager to learn about the offspring from my donation, not to meddle in their lives or supplant their parents, but just to be available. Also, I have been very successful, so I would think nothing of helping them with college tuition in a few years.

Some donors, while open to having contact with offspring, realize that sometimes there needs to be help and perhaps counseling to smooth the way if any problems arise.

Somebody would need to talk to them, what reasons they have to meet me. Certainly some independent person should be able to talk to them. I'd be open to not just meeting them but a lot more if there was an opening. I didn't think much about relations when I was a lot younger; you choose your friends and not your relations, but as I got older I changed a bit. Previously I had never thought that the possibility could arise of any chance of meeting them, but there is some chance, but not a great one. For myself, though, I'm willing to take risks in life and I have no problem about meeting new people. (Ian)

All the donors I have spoken to would never dream of initiating contact with the offspring or recipient parents. Although many donors are open to sharing information and even meeting offspring, they feel that the approach must first come from the recipient parents or the offspring.

Do sperm donors think about the infertile man? I'll leave this section with Kevin's thoughts on the matter.

I think in all this the forgotten people are actually the fathers of the children. They aren't getting much of a mention. They're probably the ones who are silently carrying a bigger burden than anyone.

Egg and embryo donors

Compared to sperm donation, egg and embryo donation is relatively recent. The first births from donated eggs or embryos only took place in the early 1980s. Originally IVF was performed with embryos which had been freshly fertilized, but it was found that if a woman could produce a number of eggs in one cycle they could all be fertilized and the resulting embryos frozen and used in later cycles. This meant that women went through fewer invasive treatments to procure eggs.

While all donation of reproductive technology has similarities, there are also some major differences. Traditionally sperm donors are paid, but in most countries egg and embryo donors are not. This has not been because of legislation but through practices set up by clinics. Although newspaper headlines have been seen around the world claiming that couples are willing to pay tens of thousands of dollars for eggs this is certainly not the norm. Reasons for the differences abound, from 'We won't get sperm donors if we don't pay them' to 'Women only want to help other women, they don't want to be paid.'

The majority of egg donation is done between relatives, usually sisters or friends. Because of the difficulty with freezing eggs, people who need donated eggs must ask someone to be a donor for them. I have recently heard of an egg bank being set up in California, but it has yet to have a successful birth. Asking a friend or relative to give her eggs is no easy matter. On the other hand, for those women who would like to donate their eggs to someone they know, making the offer is not a simple matter either, as Carolyn explains.

> My cousin couldn't produce any eggs of her own even though they said she should be able to carry a pregnancy. I thought I might be able to help her as we have a child and don't want any more. I wasn't sure how to bring up the subject with her. I didn't want her to think that I felt sorry for her, that I was pitying her. I just felt that it was the logical thing to do and it would sort of keep it in the family. I finally got up the courage to ask her and she was just blown away by the offer, they were going to advertise for a donor in the newspaper. We're going to be starting the process of donating in the next couple of months.

So, Carolyn's cousin obviously had not had the courage to ask for help from a relative. Counselors at clinics give people help in how to approach friends or relatives and bring up the subject of egg donation. They discuss many of the important issues, such as:

- the medical procedures involved, including the risks
- how to raise the subject of donation without making either party feel obligated to go through with it
- success or failure and what emotions will accompany both
- if a child results, what the relationship will be between the child and the donor
- how christenings, birthdays, Christmas and so on will be handled – will the child be singled out for special attention by the donor? (this may be fine with all concerned)
- whether the child will be told, and whether other family members and friends know.

Angela donated her eggs to her sister and she mentions some of these issues and others.

> While I was pregnant with my second child, I read an article in a magazine about a girl donating eggs to her sister and I thought this was a very special thing to do. At the time, my sister and her husband were participating in the IVF program. I did not raise the subject with them at that stage because they still had more attempts on the IVF program available to them and we were obviously all hoping for her to fall pregnant. They

continued for another 12 months without success. When the time came for their participation on the program to come to an end, I mentioned the article to my sister. I explained to her that, if it were an option in their case, I would be more than happy to donate eggs to them.

My sister, her husband, my husband, and myself discussed this quite openly and decided that it may be an option. My sister and her husband took this proposal to their doctor who decided that medically it was an option but we needed approval from the IVF clinic and extensive counseling before we could proceed.

We did have fairly extensive counseling with my sister's doctor as well as the counselor at the IVF clinic. I met with my sister's doctor on two occasions, once with my sister and once by myself. The latter occasion was to ensure that the doctor knew that I was acting of my own accord and that I was not being coerced into the situation.

The first counseling session at [the clinic] involved only my husband and myself. This was to ensure the counselor was satisfied with my reasons for donating, that I was donating of my own free will, that I was aware of the short- and long-term ramifications of being an egg donor, and that my husband was aware and comfortable with the situation. The second counseling session involved the four of us. This meeting was to ensure that we had openly discussed the pros and cons of donating and receiving donor eggs.

I went through two IVF cycles to get enough viable embryos for my sister to have the best chance of conceiving. Before I started I was warned of all the possible side effects the drugs might cause, including headaches and nausea. At no time did I suffer any side effects, although towards the end of each cycle I felt very bloated from the maturing follicles. Being an egg donor, I felt that I did not suffer from the emotional strain that most women would feel going through the IVF program. The egg pick up, performed under local anaesthetic, was slightly uncomfortable but the discomfort was outweighed by the anticipation of what the outcome would be.

At no stage throughout any of the donor procedure did I anticipate that I would be any more than a normal aunt to my sister's child. I do not think that anyone would have wished to proceed with the donation if I anticipated any more than this. My sister had a six-month waiting period before the embryos could be transferred to her. This was to ensure that all of my blood tests were clear. During this time I became pregnant with my third child. By the end of the six months I certainly had no emotional ties to the embryos that were to be transferred.

Even now, when my nephew is four years old, I feel that our relationship is that of a close extended family which includes all of my other nieces and nephews and nothing peculiar just to him. Every now and again I do stop and think that he is truly a miracle child, but this is purely a view of the wonders of modern medicine not from any emotional ties to him.

When my sister and I were going through the egg donor process, it was quite common knowledge among all of our families as well as many of our friends. There was never any secrecy about the process we were going through. At the time everyone was very supportive and very happy that my sister and her husband were being given another chance to conceive a child. Many people are obviously aware of how he was conceived and, although this is not generally discussed, the situation is very open if the subject arises.

My nephew is not fully aware of how he was conceived, as this would be very difficult to discuss with any four-year-old. He has asked his parents why he doesn't have any brothers or sisters. My sister explained to him that they had trouble having him and needed to have help from the doctors and from me. My sister and her husband plan to be very open and forthcoming about how he was conceived.

In countries like Australia many egg and embryo donors have increasingly wanted to avoid being in a totally anonymous position. They have been asking doctors to only give their eggs or embryos to couples who would like to share information. Perhaps this is coming about because most egg and embryo donors already have their own children and this can bring with it a clearer understanding of the realities of donation and what it might mean for the child created.

A friend of mine was going through IVF treatment; I saw the pain she was feeling. I already had two children and wanted to be able to help her. After four tries of IVF my friend became pregnant and had a beautiful baby girl. I still felt like it would be good to help someone so I contacted the clinic where my friend had gone.

I went in to see the counselor and we discussed things like sharing of information. I told her that I only wanted to donate to a couple who would tell the child about me. I went away and thought it all over, and my husband and I decided that I would go ahead with donating my eggs providing the clinic could find a couple who would tell their child about me and would be prepared to share information.

I've now been in hospital twice to donate to a couple and on the second try they conceived and are now about seven months pregnant. I already know a little bit about them and they know a bit about me. Hopefully in future we'll be able to swap letters or photos, and maybe one day our families can meet. (Lynda)

Whether or not to be an embryo donor is a question faced by thousands of people every year. A great many who go through IVF cycles will end up having frozen embryos in storage when they complete their families and are left with the decision of whether to donate these excess embryos or allow them to succumb (to die).

Chris and her husband, Ray, were in this situation after they had completed their family and were left with ten embryos in storage.

The two-year extension we already applied for is due to expire once again so we received a letter from our clinic asking us to make a decision. The options are as follows: commence a programme, donate the embryos, allow them to succumb, or apply for an extension of storage time. Yes, we know we could apply for yet another extension on the grounds that I need further time to consider the fate of the embryos but this is just delaying our situation. We received this letter a month ago and we know we do not wish to extend our family. This leaves us to consider the other options, which is why I know I have been avoiding this. As a couple we know it is time to move on.

To my husband it is simple; somebody helped him and us, for which he is extremely grateful, so why not give the embryos a chance to help others. After all, any couple who needs these embryos should be given that last chance to be able to experience parenthood, something that he himself enjoys to the fullest. This brings me to consider why would a couple choose embryos and not eggs? What kind of couple would seek these embryos? In my mind I knew I needed to consider these questions.

Obviously this couple would have been through much invasive treatments and could have one or more of the following reasons – early menopause, many failed cycles due to the quality of their own eggs, endometriosis, combined infertility problems – or for genetic reasons this couple may have been advised to not consider having their own genetic child. Donated embryos would be their final option.

For some, the donation of unused embryos would be quite simple and straightforward, as it was for Ray, but for others donation has to be more thoroughly thought out. Chris considered as many of the issues as she could.

> For me there are many more issues to consider than helping another couple. First, I consider our children. Thinking of my son, what are the odds that he may meet and form a relationship with a half-sibling? He has his donor's children to consider, then the offspring of the couples who used his donor's sperm, then, as well, any offspring created by these extra embryos. Then my daughter, these would be her full siblings; she also runs the same possibility of forming a relationship with a sibling. For her, if these embryos are donated, it could even be a full sibling she might meet. How will she feel, simply just knowing she has full siblings out there? Maybe angry. Is it worth trying to cope with all this to help someone else?
>
> I worried about the fact that we would have been double donating, on behalf of a sperm donor who most likely would not even know his sperm was used for an IVF cycle. I feel this is something they should always be informed of and give consent to before the IVF procedure, as [freezing embryos] enables lives to be kept in limbo and many more offspring to be created from one donor.
>
> Four months have passed since this script was started, I feel I can now sit and finish this, telling you the final outcome.
>
> I chose an outside counselor, not the one associated with my clinic. This was for no other reason than that I felt I personally needed to take myself out of the clinic environment where I had received my treatment. This enabled me to concentrate on what was best for our family, to stop putting everybody's needs first and concentrate on what was best for me. Something I was not used to doing.
>
> I also decided I needed to go to this session of counseling alone. I needed to work through my own feelings first and then if necessary my husband would attend another with me. Although my husband tried to understand and I knew he supported me, I still felt so alone. I tried to consider why I felt so alone. I came up with the following: did I want to feel like this, was I pushing the people that cared for me away? At one stage I remember feeling anger at the clinic for creating so many excess embryos and so enabling this problem to exist. I now know these actions and feelings were all because I was grieving. Like all couples, we were given the chance to make the decisions every step of the way through this cycle of IVF.

Part of the process in getting over this grief was that no matter what choice I made, whether donating or allowing these embryos to succumb, I was also accepting that I would have no further children, although I myself remain fertile. This grief was simply myself excepting my choice that my reproductive life was over. No matter how much infertility treatment you encounter and how much success, I now believe one of the hardest decisions is to know when to 'stop and move on.'

I decided we could not donate these embryos. I did not worry about the offspring searching for us one day. My concerns were simply that I knew I could not personally live life without thinking about the offspring created, without walking down the street wondering if that child could be one of mine. With that fact alone I knew it wasn't something I could do. It simply did not feel right for me to donate but it also did not feel right for me to leave these embryos in the laboratory to succumb, which is why we decided to collect them.

This decision was a very brave and well thought out one. In the short term it probably would have been so much easier to donate the embryos. Chris and Ray found their own personal way of closing a chapter of their lives and moving on. Once they had come to this decision they made an appointment to go to the clinic.

Our family went in together one Sunday morning to pick up the embryos. Our son was told what was happening. We told our son, 'Mummy may be a little sad. Mum and Dad have two beautiful children and are very happy with their family size, so are unable to use these embryos. So we need to pick them up from the hospital and put them to rest in our garden.' His answer was, 'Wow, Mum, ten's a lot of children, plus us, that's twelve. You can't have that many children.' Both children seemed very sensitive to the situation. Our little girl seemed to sense something important that involved us all was happening.

The clinic was very accommodating to our needs. I went into the area where the embryos were stored and watched while the embryologist removed them from the nitrogen tank. I checked my details with her. The five tiny straws, each containing two embryos, were handed over to me. I asked if I could look under a microscope at one of these straws. This was an important request of mine and one that was immediately granted, without questioning.

On driving home, I remember feeling relieved, but sad and withdrawn. The children were full of questions. They asked me if they could hold these straws and take a look. Their questions were answered with honesty. They both sensed they needed to be gentle and caring with these embryos. My son's understanding amazed me, as even at nine he commented that 'If one of these embryos were used instead of the ones that the staff did choose, we wouldn't be here today Mum.' My answer to this was, 'Well, Dad and I are so happy you both are.'

On returning home we spent some time together, and by late afternoon we had decided it was time to place them in the special place in our garden, a quiet little place the children had chosen, by their fishpond, surrounded by gnomes and other garden ornaments, and overlooking their play area.

The months have passed and, as we don't mention this event, we were surprised last weekend that our youngest (while playing and swinging happily on her swing) should comment, 'Our straws have gone to heaven, Daddy.'

Kathryn and her husband Paul have two daughters. Their eldest, Kaelyn, is from open adoption and Laura is a result of embryo donation from a couple who themselves used donated eggs to create the embryos. Kathryn's story is somewhat unusual and complicated, but will probably become a more common scenario as larger numbers of people tackle the issue of what to do with embryos in storage.

Laura's donors had 12 surplus embryos that they donated to the clinic for use by another infertile couple...which was us! We only thawed seven of them and were successful getting pregnant with Laura. So we had five remaining frozen embryos. I worked with the clinic for a couple of years trying to have them identify another couple who wanted to use the remaining embryos and would be willing to have some limited openness with us if a baby resulted. That matching process was never successful for many reasons, some still unclear. Of course, the standard protocol of the clinic was for embryo donations to be anonymous, so that may have been a factor although, if so, that was never directly discussed as a reason why no match could be located. (For clarification, by anonymous, I mean no identifying info. We received many pages of medical info, traits, likes/dislikes, etc. for both sperm donor and egg donor).

So, in early 1999, Paul and I attempted to find our own couple to use them. We met with two couples we had met through an adoption symposium in January, but simultaneously we discovered that a niece of Paul's and her husband were having major issues getting pregnant (with both female and male issues). The four of us were excited to move forward. However, contact with our clinic disclosed major problems. The clinic had been purchased by a major healthcare group from another state and their legal people became involved. They put the embryos into what I call 'legal limbo,' being unwilling to release them and not being willing to use them either! To make a long story short, we were forced to hire an attorney to get ownership of the embryos. The donor couple supported our claim and we three couples petitioned the clinic to release them to us for Paul's niece to use. The whole process took six months, but we won and physically moved them to another clinic. In the meantime Paul's niece became pregnant naturally.

The original protocols that the clinic wanted us to sign kept everything anonymous. We were able to have them make a modification for us to change the language to read shared identification if both parties (us and the donor couple) were agreeable. After a year of pushing I was able (through the clinic counselor) to have the donors agree to receive a letter from us, which was mailed by the clinic. After five months they wrote to us and shared their name, address and story. My main point was always that the girls (they had a daughter, too, sixteen months older than ours) had the right to meet some day and develop a relationship if they chose. Obviously, biologically they are full siblings.

With our situation there are other 'layers to the onion'…the donor couple had used a donor egg, so we have a double donation situation. We have a lot of information on the egg donor but not her identity. At this point I have not pursued communication with her. Also, there are still five remaining frozen embryos that Paul and I are currently working with the clinic to donate to another infertile couple. We want to assure openness up front if a successful pregnancy occurs.

6

Telling Others

The discovery of infertility can come as a huge shock that is hard to bear in isolation. Yet isolated is how many people feel who follow the path of donor conception. This form of infertility treatment is not an open book. It is not easy to broach this subject with others, but many feel the need for support from relatives and friends, sometimes just a shoulder to cry on and a listening ear. Some also feel the need to get things out in the open so that there are no secrets. But the big question remains, how will people react if they are told?

Steven and Catherine were very worried about how their relatives and friends would react to their using donor insemination. They worried, just like many others, that people would not understand what they were going through; that people might reject the choice of donor conception and then where would that leave them?

> My family are quite religious and DI is not an accepted idea in the Catholic Church. After putting forward the problems which could occur they saw it from our side and were then completely behind us. Older members of my family said things like, 'It isn't really right but it's the only option,' or, 'It is none of our business but good luck to them.'
>
> Steven's parents were very detached, not interested really, but they are like this with all their grandchildren so I don't think that the DI made any difference to them. One of his brothers and his sister-in-law have been really interested and positive. His sister feels embarrassed to discuss any of it with us and really pretends nothing has occurred. My girlfriends were amazing. One of my old flat mates has now donated eggs; she was so relieved to have had her children easily and wanted to give this chance to someone else. We had some beautiful letters from friends giving us support.

In my own experience, I felt the need to tell everyone. My husband and I had no family close by. Relatives were interstate or overseas, so we told friends. I think, as with many others, our initial reason for telling others was to get support; to be able to talk it over with someone who was not grieving as we were. I have always felt better from talking through my feelings and I know now that had I kept all my thoughts and feelings inside it would have been even more difficult to bear.

When people start going beyond their circle of very close friends and relatives, and disclosing their use of donor conception, it is possible for them to lose control over who knows. Some people such as, Janet and Julian, have thought this over and decided to be very careful about whom they tell.

> We told Julian's five brothers and sisters, his parents, my brother and sister and parents, and probably three couples who were close friends. I also told another three close girlfriends so we did talk to people and we found that the couples who had children were the most understanding.
>
> I think there is a bit of an attitude, especially in our rural area, that it's always the woman who has the fertility problems. For that reason, people in our immediate community don't know. It could make it hard for Julian if people knew; it's a very blokey kind of a community. Often people are very surprised when they hear about male infertility. Julian's mum was quite shocked, I think she had really felt that there was something wrong with me. Later she thought that maybe when she was pregnant with Julian she took a tablet, or maybe she was unwell or not eating properly, and that caused the infertility. She will still refer to it from time to time, and I think she would really like to know what caused Julian's infertility, but we don't know. (Janet)
>
> I could never imagine going to the pub with other friends and saying, 'Listen fellas, while we're on the subject, I'm infertile.' I just couldn't do it; they'd have the biggest laugh. Well, they probably wouldn't, but you'd feel like they'd laugh. A couple of days after I found out I was infertile the first person I told was my best friend, a fellow who lived just down the road. I told my friend because I could trust him and he's been a close friend for a lot of years. It was just comforting to tell someone about it, and he was pretty good about it. But he said the same thing my dad said: 'Don't worry about it, she'll be right, one day they'll be able to fix it.' It would be good if you could really talk about it. (Julian)

Our experience of talking to others, even beyond close friends, has been overwhelmingly positive – no one has recoiled in horror or said that we shouldn't do it. We have had a huge amount of curiosity – does it involve IVF, who are the donors, do you get to choose the donor, are you going to tell your child, can you meet the donor? Of course there have been some who obviously felt that they couldn't ask questions about it and we have never forced information on these people, but if someone has asked us a question we have always tried to answer it.

Many others have also had positive experiences.

> We told my immediate family when we went on the program and we told Paul's immediate family after Jake was born. We didn't have any negative feedback at all. One of my sisters said, 'I've watched people go through IVF programs and thought, I wonder why Barbara doesn't try that?' but didn't think it was her business to say anything to me. Paul's family, they said, 'Well, he's still our grandchild.' That's all we've told except for the doctors. Paul strongly believes that it's nobody else's business. (Barbara)

> We told Nicholas's parents first. Initially they were quite shocked, and his mother, I think, felt dreadful, as though in some way she'd done something. It's unexplained infertility, no apparent reason for it at all, and his brothers have both been checked and they're fine.
>
> Nicholas's parents are intelligent people, they were able to deal with their shock but it was quite a bombshell coming out of the blue. They were very concerned and anxious to help him as much as possible.
>
> Initially we talked to very close family like our parents but our intention all along was to gradually tell our close friends and family. We've only told people who we feel need to know. Though sometimes I have met people who I don't know and I've disclosed information to them because it seemed appropriate, but I don't tell mutual friends unless I have first talked to Nicholas about how he feels. Basically, we have told anyone who will know our child because we want the child to grow up feeling that their circumstances are quite normal. If they happened to ask that person about their background, that person would have answers for them. (Mary)

While those who cannot have their own biological children grieve the loss of genetic continuance, this loss will also affect others. The infertile person's parents may never have their own genetic grandchild, siblings their own genetic nephews or nieces. These relatives may also be grieving. Cathy talks about how this affected her family.

> I told my siblings the day I told them I was pregnant. I had been through IVF the year before and had not told them until after it was over and it had failed. This second time, I simply told them that my husband and I were 'doing the baby thing again.' They only know that it is donor ovum, they do not know that we also used donor sperm mixed with my husband's sperm.
>
> My siblings, with whom I am very close, did not take the information well. I told them on the phone, so I couldn't get a visual reaction, but I could tell they were confused by the information. They didn't know how to respond. They were happy for me, but I think very disappointed that my child 'wouldn't be related' to them. In fact, my brother said, 'Oh, then I guess my sons won't have a cousin after all.' I think he immediately regretted saying that, but it just came out before he had a chance to think how hurtful it was.
>
> I think now, after three months, they are accepting it a little better, but they are very disappointed that they are not getting a blood-related niece or nephew. One sister said, 'Gee, we won't get to see who it looks like–it won't have any of our family's features.'
>
> Part of the pain I felt was their disappointment. Having a child should be a celebration, but for them, the news was a huge let-down. If I had it to do over again, I don't think I would tell them. Or maybe well after the children were born, after they had all bonded with them. Then the information, I think, would not have been so traumatic for them, and perhaps would have been even inconsequential at that point.
>
> We did not tell my husband's parents about anything donor related. They just think we used some fertility drugs. They're in their eighties and we thought that it just wouldn't help them to know.
>
> Friends, the few that we have told, have been much more open to the news than my family. Only three know the whole story, including the donor sperm. They are very supportive and have bent over backwards to be helpful.

It is without question easier for most women to talk about infertility than it is for men. I think my husband was lucky because, for some unexplained reason, he could and still does tell others about his infertility. His attitude from the outset has been, 'If others don't like it, it's their problem.' But in a society where male infertility is still a relatively closed subject, it is under-standable that many men will have some reticence about the subject.

As my husband and I went further and further down the DI path in the late 1980s we both realized how infrequently donor conception was talked about and how little knowledge there was about it in the community. This became another reason for us to talk about it; we both felt that if we were open about how we were conceiving our children then it might help others in the same situation. We also felt that it could help the wider community to a better understanding of infertility in general and donor conception in particular.

We took this one step further when trying to conceive our second child. The clinic we were attending asked for a couple who would be willing to do media interviews in order to attract more sperm donors. We did numerous TV and newspaper interviews and talked about having a child by DI and how we would tell our children how they were conceived. We, along with others, have continued this work through the DCSG in Australia and we feel that we have gone someway to increasing community knowledge of donor conception.

While many married couples can choose who they tell about using donor conception, single women and lesbian couples are inevitably going to be asked questions about who the father of the child is. Most choose to be very upfront from the beginning, as did Deborah, Susan, and Christina.

> My family knows, everyone knows. The thing is I've never slept around and my mother has told everyone how I conceived this child because she doesn't want people to think that I just went out and had a one-night stand.
>
> My cousin from England came and stayed with me for two weeks and came to see the ultrasound. My other cousin in Melbourne said that if she can she's going to be here for the birth. It surprised the hell out of me because my cousins are about fifteen years older than me. This baby is bringing us closer as a family. (Deborah)

> I am being very open about this procedure. In fact, with my last preg-nancy, I became so ill with morning sickness that I had to let my adminis-trator in on what was going on with me. I live in a conservative commu-nity and it is known that I am a single woman. I just explained my circum-stances as being one of high-tech pre-natal adoption. With the last preg-nancy, this was only half true, in that I had adopted only the sperm. With

my next pregnancy (using both donor sperm and eggs), adoption is the most accurate description anyone could come up with. While I won't be explaining the nature of my conception to my third and fourth grade students, I will be open about it with their parents, my fellow staff members, and the community at large. (Susan)

I have spoken openly and freely with all my family, including my father, mother, and stepfather, three female siblings, and many, many friends both straight and gay. Most of their reactions have been wonderful and excited. My three sisters all had similar reactions at first. They were all brought up by my mother and I by my father. To varying degrees they were very concerned that my child would not know or have the nurturing of a father. They wondered what kind of baggage and issues the child might have to carry. Also, did I really have the right to have a child if I had chosen to be a lesbian?

Since that time, which is quite a few years ago now, they have really done a lot of soul searching and discussion with their own friends and people they have met and are really happy about the idea, but it has taken much searching, analyzing and love on their part to really come to terms with the whole thing. I must say all of my sisters have always said no matter how they feel intellectually about me having a child they would always accept him or her into our family with love. I love them dearly for being so honest and now accepting. I feel so lucky for both my partner and me and any children that are to come. My mother and father, who are divorced but have partners, are both so supportive and wonderful; they can't wait for their precious grandchild to be born. (Christina)

Jane and her partner took some time to decide to tell their family but opted to do it before the conception.

I was concerned about us telling our parents. My parents took long enough to accept the fact that I am in a relationship with another woman. We decided we had to tell them fairly early. We never wanted to get that question, 'Why didn't you tell us before?'

As Jane mentions, apart from the decision of who to tell there is also the decision of when to tell. A number of years ago I talked to a man who, with his wife, because of his genetic condition was trying to conceive their child using donor insemination. They decided to tell their friends and relatives even before they commenced on a program. He realized that people they knew might be concerned that any child they conceived would also have his genetic condition. They told everyone they were using donated sperm so they would not worry that a child would inherit the husband's health problems.

Glenda, a single woman, told her sister and parents before she began on a program, and she explains how she went about telling them.

> When the clinic told me that I could start on the DI program at any time I told my parents. I didn't want them to find out when I was pregnant and to take it badly when it should be a time of celebration. I wanted to give them enough time to get used to the idea before it actually happened.
>
> I didn't know what to say. I'd been thinking for a couple of days how to say it and it still didn't come out the way I thought it would. I'd recently taken a day off work; my father had asked if I was sick and I'd said yes. So when I went to tell them I said, 'You know when you rang and I said I was sick, well I wasn't actually sick, I went to a clinic to see if I can have a baby.' I just came out and told them what I was doing. They asked how it worked and things like that. The most amazing part of it was they took it so well. They were surprised, of course, because it had never happened in our family or circle of friends before.
>
> I had the biggest headache before I got there, and then afterwards I thought, 'Thank God, it's all right.' I had already talked to my sister at this stage and she said that Mum and Dad could go and talk to her about it if they were having a hard time with it, if they wanted to bring up things that I might not want to hear, then there was someone they could go and talk to.

The number of families bringing their own donors to a clinic is increasing in many areas. Using a known donor brings with it some different issues, such as: if we tell people who the donor is, will they be forever comparing our child to the donor, will they be checking out how the donor interacts with the child?

Lynette and her husband have kept private the knowledge that they used a known donor, and she explains why.

> There's a difference between privacy and secrecy. I am generally a fairly private person, so while our children know about their origins, and it's discussed openly at home, and with the doctor and those who need to know, we haven't told our families or most of our friends. Some know that the children were born by donor conception, but we haven't felt comfortable about telling people who the donor is. I guess its because we

don't need the pressure of having to deal with their reactions. Most people probably wouldn't believe that our son is not biologically linked to his dad anyway.

So, I guess there's a sense of living a lie to other people, but then it's not their business. The children know, and that's the main thing. If they choose to tell other people as they get older then that's their prerogative and we'll accept that. In the meantime, they have a positive relationship with the man who helped to make them. They are growing up with a half-brother (our donor's son) who also knows why they're special.

Andrew and Bronwyn have also told friends and family how they conceived their daughter but not who the donor is.

The one who had the hardest time adjusting was my wife's mother. A widow, she felt very strongly the sense of loss that there would be no genetic link to the child. I predicted that this would change when she held the baby in her arms. I was right. She is a doting and very proud grandmother. Only Bronwyn's mother knows the identity of our donor. We did not tell her, she worked it out for herself. She wrote the donor a beautiful letter thanking her and telling her how much happiness the donor's generosity had brought her.

The decision about who else should know how a child was conceived goes beyond family and friends. Do people tell their obstetrician, paediatrician, family doctor, or even their child's teachers? One of the common questions that a doctor will ask is, 'Is there a family history of…?' Parents have to make a decision about whether to tell that doctor about their child's conception because in most cases they will know very little about the medical history of the donor. In our case, we have been told that there is nothing of significance in the medical histories of our children's three donors. But what does that mean? We also know that none of them has given any updated medical information to the clinic. Does that mean that their families are all healthy or just that they have never thought to tell the clinic that they now know that a number of their close relatives have had heart disease or bowel cancer, for example? For this reason, we felt that we should tell our family doctor that we know virtually nothing about the donor's medical history. We felt that this knowledge could aid in decisions he makes about any medical tests our children might need.

As donor-conceived children grow there could be others that might need to know and parents will have to make decisions about this as time goes on. Rob decided that he should tell his son's teachers.

> To protect Jack we even told his teachers. We didn't want little rumours starting in the schoolyard. Kids obviously discuss how children are conceived and we wanted the teachers to be aware of it. I think for a lot of them it was quite novel, they quite nonchalantly said, 'Oh right, OK,' but deep down you can see their mind ticking over and thinking, 'Oh, gosh.'

We also chose to tell our children's teachers for the same reason. Our son Callum was for quite a while convinced that all parents had to go to a hospital to get sperm to conceive a child, and we certainly didn't want a playground dispute over where babies come from. Our children's teachers have been very respectful of our sharing this information with them, and the playground dispute that we feared never eventuated.

7

Treatment, Pregnancy, and Birth

Starting treatment with donor conception is usually a time of very mixed emotions. Great hope that now the dreams of a child may be finally realized, but also fear: how will we cope with treatment both physically and emotionally, will it be successful, what if it doesn't work?

Being on an infertility program has been likened to riding a roller-coaster. The upsurge of hope when you begin the lead up to insemination, egg pick up, or embryo transfer. The extreme nervousness when that day arrives. Then the waiting period, pregnant or not? This is like being poised at the top of the roller-coaster. After that, for so many people it's a downward rush into sadness: it didn't work.

The journey to conceive our first son took about a year from the time we started on our first treatment cycle. For some, this will seem a long time but for others a year is a drop in the ocean. To be honest, I was not a nice person a lot of the time when I was trying to conceive. I would, at various times, be sad, angry, desperate, and furious at the seeming unfairness of it all. I did not accept at all well, the upsetting of my plans to have a family. I have, of course, found since then that my reactions were not that unusual and probably for the most part quite normal given the circumstances.

> There were emotional traumas with trying to have a baby, like Barbara, her temper was incredible. All the way through, every couple of weeks, her temper was changing. That was the hardest thing for me to handle, her spitting the dummy all the time. (Paul)

Donor insemination, when used for treating male infertility, brings with it a special set of circumstances. Women are undergoing medical treatment for what is a male problem. Men can feel guilty for putting their wives 'through infertility treatment.' Kate explains how her husband John felt when they were trying DI.

> I worked throughout it all and I felt that I needed to work because it was good for me mentally to relieve the stress of the treatments. For those first two or three years John was devastated. He would say, 'I've got the problem and you've got to have all these injections, you've got to have the operations, it's crazy.' A lot of the time I had my injections at home. John gave me the injections and at first he didn't cope well and would say, 'Not only do you have to go through all the pain, now I'm giving you more with these injections.' But I would say, 'No, you're helping me because it means I don't have to go into the clinic.' I think that's probably why our society doesn't see male infertility as being a real issue, because the woman is still the one who has to go through all the treatment.

There is one area of DI that is very rarely talked about and that is how couples deal with the fact that the woman is being inseminated by another man's sperm, usually an unknown person. Personally, at the time of treatment, it was no more to me than another medical procedure that would hopefully give me a child. Many others feel the same way but for some it is not so easy to deal with, as Joe describes.

> I hated it. When Marie went for treatment I felt like she was off having an affair. Of course I never told her that, I kept it to myself. We wanted a child; there wasn't any other choice. When the baby was born I kept looking at her to see if there might be something that wasn't from Marie's family, something that had to have come from the donor. Over the years I've gradually come to feel better about things. Kristy's four now and we think we might start telling her soon about the special way she came into the world.

As was discussed in Chapter 4 *Choosing a Donor* it was a practice some years ago for some doctors to mix the semen of the donor and the husband in order to disguise paternity. In most countries this practice is now either illegal or considered to be unethical, but it does still occur, as Cathy describes.

> The ova were harvested on a Sunday, and by that evening we knew that my husband's sperm had only barely survived the freeze. Out of three phials of frozen sperm (it had been extracted from the epididymus a year earlier and was not 'mature' sperm) only nine sperm had any motility at

all. The embryologist said the sperm did not look great, and recommended that we use donor sperm for the remainder of the 20 ovum. (We had donor sperm selected in case Jim's sperm didn't survive the freeze). All this information came to us via the telephone. The embryologist is in the lab, I'm at home, and my husband is a thousand miles away in a hotel room on a business trip. I had the difficult task of calling him to tell him the news.

On the phone, my husband and I decided to go with the embryologist's decision. Then we waited for the news of how the embryos did. We would know the next morning, a Monday.

Monday came. The embryologist called and said that only two of the nine embryos of my husband's sperm began the dividing process. All of the eleven donor sperm embryos were doing well. Again, I had to call my husband between business meetings with this news. He was devastated, but had to turn around and continue with all-day meetings.

We waited and watched. Wednesday came, the day of the transfer. My husband and I were both glum. We met with the embryologist, and he suggested we use the two embryos of my husband's sperm (which were not doing well at all, one was at a two-cell stage and the other only at the one-cell stage) and to use three of the donor sperm embryos. I was thinking, five? Isn't that a bit high?

Clearly, the embryologist felt that my husband's embryos would not make it. At this clinic, the typical number of donor ovum embryos transferred to a woman my age (forty-four) was three.

Jim and I were given 10, maybe 15 minutes to discuss this. Not enough time to make this kind of difficult and life-changing decision. I was in a state of shock and not at all able to think clearly. My whole reason for using donor ovum was so that at least my husband could have a shot at having a child of his own, and now the whole thing had gotten too weird. I fought the urge to scream out that if they weren't my husband's, I didn't want them at all. That is how I truly felt. But we had spent so much money… so I kept quiet. Jim and I decided yes: his two, and only two of the donor sperm.

Then we went into the transfer room, the nurse got me all prepared, then the doctor came in. (This was the first time we had seen the doctor in several weeks). He asked, 'So, how many are we transferring today?' We said four. He looked angry and almost yelling, demanded, 'Only four? You do want to get pregnant, don't you?'

I felt bullied. Meekly I said, 'Well, I suppose we can reduce if there are too many.' The doctor blurted out, 'None of my patients has ever reduced, even if they have three!' Here I was, lying on the table, bladder full, legs in stirrups, the most vulnerable position a woman can be in. I felt powerless. We agreed to the doctor's wishes.

I knew I was pregnant before the results were in. I was terrified from then until the first ultrasound that all five of them were growing. My Human Chorionic Gonadotrophin (HCG) level was off the charts. So I was very relieved to find they were only twins. *Only twins*?! This was crazy, I didn't want twins. So now I'm pregnant, but with whose sperm?

I'm pretty angry, as you can tell. I think the doctor wanted to ensure a pregnancy just to make his statistics look good. I really don't feel he had our best interests at heart.

The quest for a child may take a very long time and for some couples there may come a point one day when they have to sit down and decide if they will continue with treatment or stop. Andrea and Mark came to this point in their lives a few years ago, as Andrea describes.

We tried donor sperm with my eggs for about five cycles but it just wasn't working. Apparently my eggs were not very good. Even with IVF it didn't work. This was in the days before ICSI. I brought it up with Mark that I wasn't sure if I could keep going with treatment and he said he'd been thinking the same thing. We cried a lot, we'd always wanted to have children, we don't have a very big family and I had imagined me, one day, being the grandmother of numerous little grandchildren. We took a few weeks, talking about it and grieving, then we rang the clinic and said we wouldn't be coming in any more. I can't say that there aren't times when I'm not sad about it but we have a very rich and wonderful life and are involved with friends' and relatives' children.

Belinda and Michael have been trying to have a child for some time and have thought about what they will do if DI is not successful.

We both want to have children more than anything in the world. Adoption is certainly on the cards if this doesn't work, but having a child from birth and experiencing pregnancy are also things we don't want to miss out on if that's at all possible. Having now had six unsuccessful cycles, we have started talking more about this possibility, but at this stage are still hoping we will be able to have a child through DI. (Belinda)

> I don't want Belinda to miss out on the experience of pregnancy and breastfeeding and other things that go with that. However, I realize that at some point, if still unsuccessful we will have to stop treatment, and I am quite happy to consider adoption. (Michael)

Anne and Carl have a very different story about stopping treatment, as Anne relates.

> I said to my doctor, 'That's it. I can't take any more.' I had decided that I didn't want to be pregnant at forty. Childbearing was something for my twenties and thirties and it was a time to end. Three weeks later our doctor rang up and offered us some eggs. It was essentially my husband's decision. I said, 'If you want to use them that's OK and if you don't, that's fine.' He said that he wanted to use them and so we did.
>
> My husband wanted these eggs, he felt very positive about them. In fact, I sort of had feelings that it would work this time. The really bizarre thing was that these eggs were offered to two other couples before they were offered to us, and they didn't want them which is really just ridiculous as donor eggs are in such short supply. But for various reasons they just turned them down. It was from these eggs that our daughter was born.

The roller-coaster of infertility is not just reserved for the people who go through treatment. We have already mentioned the feelings of their partners, but apart from that friends and families can also be affected. They are hoping that treatment will be successful because they see the pain their friends or relatives are experiencing and they want to see that go away. But what about the donors of both egg and sperm? How do they cope with the results of their donations success or lack of it?

The majority of egg donors are known to the person they give their eggs to. They undergo a similar treatment to the infertile – injections to stimulate egg production and then egg retrieval, both of which carry risks. Women donors will invest their emotions and their bodies to help another woman achieve her dream. What happens when this doesn't work?

> I'd already had two children when my sister got married. Not long after, they started to try and have a family. It never happened. After investigations by the doctors, my sister found that she couldn't have children of her own. She was devastated. I felt terrible, but after only a few days of

thought I offered to give some of my eggs to her and her husband. I managed to produce six eggs the first time and they made four embryos. My sister had two tries at getting pregnant but nothing happened. The next time I only produced three eggs and none of them fertilized. I feel I've let my sister down, I grieve for her and for the fact that I can't seem to help her. The feeling is terrible. (Emma)

The assumption is often made that when a man donates sperm there will inevitably be children born from the donations. This isn't always the case, which can bring unexpected feelings. Greg said, 'I am disappointed that a birth has not happened as a result of my donations' and that it would be 'fantastic' to meet any offspring that might be born.

Pregnancy is the goal towards which infertile people strive. They are sometimes ill prepared for the stresses of pregnancy. Throughout treatment, many come to expect failure and loss. There are those who begin their pregnancy expecting it to fail, the birth at the end of the pregnancy is lost in the mists of the future, it is not real. Many feel that they cannot truly be fertile until they are parents, so pregnancy for them can be like living in limbo.

I remember thinking while still trying to conceive that when I finally became pregnant I would celebrate. I would cook a special dinner for Patrice and put a pair of baby booties beside his plate as a way of telling him that it had finally happened. It would be a time of celebration. When I did conceive I didn't have the exultant feeling that I had expected. The happiness that I felt was very much tinged with, 'But maybe I'll miscarry or something will happen.' I bled on and off for the first 11 weeks so never felt truly joyful.

For some parents the reality of using donated gametes starts to sink in only when they conceive.

As soon as I was pregnant and it became a reality I felt more threatened, and I didn't think that I would feel like that, but maybe it's quite a reasonable thing to feel. I had thought that when the baby was born I'd write to the donor and tell him, now I'm not sure that I could do that. I sort of console myself that I don't know what purpose that would serve, but I'd be quite happy for him to be told about the birth of the baby. (Mary)

Richard didn't want to think about the fact that they had used donor sperm to have their daughter.

In my mind it was now 'fixed.' My wife was pregnant and to the outside world nothing appeared amiss. Once my daughter was born and we got home, I burned all the non-identifying information. No one needed to know, not even my daughter.

Some parents spend the nine months worrying about possible problems: they fear miscarriage, birth defects, and the concern of many who used donated gametes or embryos – what will the child look like? Of course fertile couples also spend time imagining what their child is going to look like; will it have the husband's nose or grandma's red hair? For a couple who have used donor conception with an anonymous donor there is a big unknown.

> To be pregnant at last was my life's most wonderful experience and, apart from the toxaemia and the last two weeks in hospital before her birth, I enjoyed the nine months so much. Even though I loved what I was carrying, I had a fear that maybe it was not a baby they put inside me (I didn't have an ultrasound). A lot of people would not understand this, but I feared the seeds could have belonged to anything. After she was born I would just sit in awe looking at this beautiful baby who was really ours, but for two to three days I missed having her inside me. I also hated putting her to bed at night because I felt I'd never see her exactly the same again. (Jenny)

> I know I felt like a single mum when I was pregnant, I knew there was this person out there and I didn't fit with him but…I suppose maybe it was because I was younger. (Gwen)

> I had a lot of strange dreams with the donor's face during the pregnancy. Not a child's face, a man's face always on the baby. Maybe it was because we don't know what the donor looks like. (Vivianne)

> I had a lot of dreams while I was pregnant about having a child who was not socially acceptable in some way. In one recurring nightmare I would read that a baby should be around fifty centimetres long but I gave birth to these four tiny babies. I would have a ruler and I'd be lining them all up and together they measured fifty centimetres, and I'd be thinking, 'It's all right, it's all right, they're the right length.' It was obviously a worry that this child wasn't going to be right and somehow it would be a punishment or a result of using donor conception. I was quite concerned during

the actual pregnancy, especially when I started thinking about the issues more deeply. (Janet)

I had moments during the pregnancy where I lay in bed at night and my husband would be asleep, and I'd be thinking, 'Oh my, what have I done?' I'd occasionally think of things like what if a mix up happened in the laboratory with the eggs and the babies were very dark skinned, or with red hair and freckles, something totally opposite to my husband and me? (Vivianne)

It's not just looks that people worry about. It can be as basic as: 'Will we love this baby?' Julian was concerned about this.

While Janet was pregnant it was fantastic just that she was pregnant and we were going to have a baby. I felt we were blessed but at the same time I was just a little bit scared of what might happen. There's this baby that's not biologically mine, am I going to love it? I didn't know how I would react on seeing the child when it was born and I was just scared of that moment. When it did actually happen, when Janet had Oscar, it was fantastic. I remember I felt that I was the only father that ever had a son. From the moment I saw Oscar there was no hesitation whatsoever.

While the majority of people using donor gametes are heterosexual couples, there are growing numbers of single women using fertility programs. How do women who are by themselves cope with the stress of pregnancy without a partner?

My father came along as my birthing partner and when we started the birthing classes they went around and we introduced ourselves and I said, 'And this is my dad,' but I didn't mention that I'd used DI. It was great to see him so excited and both Mum and Dad came along to the 18-week ultrasound. They had never seen anything like it, even though they'd had their own children and six grandchildren, but as my siblings had partners they didn't go along to things like that. I think Dad's a bit of an expert on the reproductive system now.

The whole process just amazed me; I didn't realize how little I knew about my own body. For the couple of weeks before she was due I kept wondering what she would look like. It was all becoming very, very real. When she was born, she was just gorgeous. I hardly thought about having the donor sperm, it was just so overwhelming. (Glenda)

Using a known donor can have different concerns. How will the donor react when he or she sees the baby? Will they want to be a parent to the child? June did have some worries about this but overcame them because of the openness she had with her egg donor.

> I did worry about how my girlfriend would react when the babies were born and we talked about that. Her kids had always called me Auntie June because we're close. My girlfriend thought that seeing my babies might have a special feel to it but that she would feel that way about my babies anyway. A close friend of hers who was also on IVF at the time conceived just before me. My girlfriend used that quite often as a parallel. She said, 'I'm already like this with Sue's babies, and I didn't have anything to do with their conception.'

When the moment of birth arrives there can be the fear that others have mentioned. What the baby will look like. In the case of DI some parents can be happy to attribute as many of the child's characteristics to the maternal side as possible. Parents may have a hard time thinking that their child looks like the donor, someone they have never seen and cannot put a name to. I have unusual eyes; my three children, born from three different donors, also have them. Sometimes a little thought creeps up on me that I'm glad they have my eyes because then there is less of them connected to the three men who donated their sperm to create them. I feel guilty about these thoughts because my children are connected to these men; after all, they contributed 50 percent of their biological makeup. I'm sure my ambivalence about their donors is not unusual and I have a feeling that if I ever got to meet these men the fear would go away.

Once a child has been born, we can put very high expectations on ourselves as parents because of all that we have been through to get this far. I assumed that I would fall instantly in love with my children, that I would never scream at them, that I would be the perfect parent. I felt that I should be forever grateful that I had a child. Andrew explains his thoughts on this.

> Some couples start a baby for the cost of a large pizza and a bottle of red, it cost us $8000 and a ride on an emotional roller-coaster. You would have to say that we really wanted to have a child. It meant that our expectations were very high and our joy and gratitude for the birth of our daughter was extremely high. I can't, however, claim that this means I love my child much more than a 'normal' father would. I am sure that any

father who loves his child does so with full measure. Nothing prepared me for how special it would feel to have my daughter crawl across the floor and wrap her arms around my leg to be picked up. I cannot adequately describe what it feels like when she looks at me and bursts into a brilliant smile. Saying thank you does not begin to say what I feel towards a special woman and her husband, who gave us such a special gift.

The first few months after Oscar was born did not quite go the way Janet expected.

After having Oscar, I had post-natal depression and I think a lot of that was to do with the donor aspect of it and the fact that he was quite a difficult baby. My mum was really supportive, as was my maternal health centre nurse, who felt that I should have been watched more closely. She felt that the donor conception should have been seen as a factor that might pre-determine a condition like post-natal depression. I felt terribly guilty for feeling that way after wanting this child and being through so much. But I found that talking to people helped a lot, and after a while I felt that I was developing a good relationship with Oscar and it all gradually changed.

Barbara had quite high expectations of herself as a parent.

There are many occasions when you think that you've got to be better than the average mother and he's got to be a better child. Sometimes I feel like standing on a mountain and shouting, 'He is the most special boy in the world and no one knows what it's like to have gone through what we did to have this special baby and aren't we lucky to have our Jake.'

8

To Tell or Not to Tell

The question that must inevitably be answered by all people who use donor conception is, 'Should we tell our child how they were conceived?'

For decades, the vast majority of people followed the direction given to them by their doctors, 'Do not tell,' as Evelyn and Anne describe.

> Our doctor said that if we conceived there was no need to tell our children, there was no need for them to ever know. That was a long time ago, 27 years ago. We agreed with it in those days, I mean we were pretty ignorant then. It was never suggested that the child might need to know. We never even thought past having the child. (Evelyn)

> We asked the doctor what we should tell our child and what did other people tell their children? He said that most people 'didn't say anything,' so we didn't say anything except to each other for the first three years of Mae's life. It felt like there was an enormous burden hanging over us. (Anne)

When we look back the twenty or so years ago that Evelyn and Anne are talking about it was the general understanding of the time that children born of donated gametes did not need to know how they were conceived. True openness in adoption was only just beginning, and very few people were making any link between adoption and donor conception.

It is very hard to go against a tide of people, starting from the doctor, all saying that the child does not need to know, that it's best not to tell. At the beginning, it seems easiest to go with the flow, as Gwen describes.

> We wanted the donor's blood group matched to my husband's in case we didn't tell them. I was paranoid about them finding out at school or something; you know when they do their little blood tests in high school

(biology). I wanted to tell them. I always thought that it wasn't fair not to tell them, but the doctor didn't, he said, 'You don't have to, the child doesn't have to know, pretend like it's your husband's.' I couldn't pretend it was. My husband wasn't so sure so we just played it safe. I knew what I wanted but he wasn't quite ready. His family didn't give much support, it was this big pretend thing, pretend it's Paul's, and I couldn't.

Although people like those above initially followed the advice given by their doctors, over time it became something that they could not live with, as Jenny describes.

The doctor told us then (18 years ago) to keep the AI completely private and no one, including the child, would ever know. He had me feeling that in time we'd forget how we'd conceived. I can't remember when I started to feel they should be told, but I think it was when they were very young. I didn't want this secret we were frightened to talk about near them, but I also felt it was unfair that someone else knew and they didn't. As time went by, I felt it was their right as individuals to know and I began wondering when to tell them.

There have always been parents like Jenny who have decided that concealing the truth was not for them. Leonie's eldest child is now eighteen and Leonie used her own personal experiences to come to a decision, along with her husband, about telling their daughter of her conception.

When I was pregnant with Geraldine, I was using the Freedom of Information Act, trying to get my own information about being a state ward from the Victorian Government. Within a month of Geraldine being born, I started to ask myself questions about my own identity and would Geraldine feel the same way about her identity. Warren and I talked about whether to keep it a secret or not. Warren felt that nobody else should know before the children were told, but I went ahead and told some friends. Warren was very upset and angry about that. I needed people to talk to, but he didn't want anyone else to know at that stage.

We realized there was a cloud hanging over us, a big weight on our shoulders. We had to tell. I really had lots of reservations about telling in some sense. Was I trying to make myself happier by unburdening my stuff about this and then burdening my child? But then, I thought, it doesn't have to be a burden for her, it's the way you tell them, it's what you do with that information, if people are supportive of their children it doesn't have to be a burden.

Richard felt that the only way he could father his child was to keep the fact that they used DI a complete secret; but over time, he came to change his mind.

> I found that I could not forget about the treatment, even though I tried to pretend that it had not happened. Initially, if I was to see the children as my own, I had to forget about the donor. Over time, I found myself confiding to others about the DI treatments. We talked a lot at home about keeping secrets and decided that ultimately they could be detrimental and destructive to our marriage and our future relationships with our children. What if they found out by chance when they were older, through changes in legislation or in a heated argument? Nothing destroys a loving family more quickly than loss of trust. We decide that we could not chance it, we would have to tell them. If they were to know of their origins it would have to be while they were young. But how? We could only discuss matters between ourselves up to a point. We did not know anyone who had adult DI children and my greatest fear was that I would be rejected by my children in favour of, as I saw it, their 'real' father. I said to Heather many times, 'You will always be their mother.' I felt I was jeopardizing my relationship, but my wife had nothing to lose.
>
> I was watching a commercial on TV one night about safe sex. It featured a beer mat, on one side it had a picture of a sperm and on the other side it said, 'It takes more than this to be a father.' Immediately it struck home to me that fatherhood was, and is, the day-to-day caring for and supporting, watching them grow up. This was the answer I had been looking for, though we still were not sure where to begin telling them and how.

A great many people have asked me why Patrice and I decided to tell our children. Both of us grew up in homes where things were not very open. Major events happened in our lives with little or no discussion, no opportunity for us to understand what was going on. Before we conceived our children by donor insemination we both agreed to tell them how they were conceived. At the time we did not really discuss it, we just knew it was the right thing to do.

We realized only years later why we had come to this decision. For us, living in openness and honesty is the healthy way for our family to be.

Keeping knowledge as important as biological identity from our children would have been like a millstone around out necks. Our children are growing up knowing how they were conceived and, for us, telling them the truth was a measure of our respect for them as individual human beings.

I remember some time ago reading a book which posed the question, 'If a person never knows the truth how can they be harmed?' Secrets are not quite as simple as that. Living with a secret can be extremely hard. To keep the secret of a child's conception means that there will always be a certain division in the family. On one side there will be those that know the secret and on the other those, most especially the child, who don't.

If parents keep a secret from their own children, it will mean that there has to be distance between them. There will be certain areas of conversation that they may feel uncomfortable with; certain topics that will feel 'too close to home.' Children can be very sensitive to an adult's unease about a subject. Tim feels that not telling his children the truth would inevitably have an impact on his relationship with them.

> A lot of my friends don't even know what happened to me so I know that if you keep things back from people it's amazing how it can permeate right through a relationship. I know that in a lot of my male relationships there's a certain amount of distance and I'm sure a lot of it comes from not telling them everything about me. I know, taking that as a parallel, with children there is no way you could not tell your child about their conception. It would just show through the relationship and I would be more fearful of destroying the relationship than I would be of letting them know.

If parents have told their children about their conception this means they do not have to fear certain subjects that may come up for discussion within the family. If their children want to talk about conception in general or their own in particular, there are no barriers.

I look on telling my children in a way that some people might find rather confronting. If my husband and I had let our children believe that they were biologically related to both of us, then we would be letting them believe something that is not true, letting them believe that they are someone other than who they really are. I remember, years ago, watching a television show where an adult who was conceived by donor insemination talked about finding out the truth of his conception. He said he had worked hard for many years building his identity (as all children do as they grow), but when he was told that he was conceived from a donor and was not biologically related to his father he had to start building all over again. Some parents who have not told their children while they are young may look on this as a good reason never to tell their older children. But no, although I feel it is preferable for children to be told at a young age, those donor-conceived adults who were told later in life still feel that they are better off knowing. For many it answers questions that have gone unanswered for years, and they feel it is their right to know and knowing has brought about a new basis for their relationships with their parents.

Today the number of parents telling their children is growing, and there can be many different reasons why these parents are open with their children. Some, like Carl and Paul, realize that in today's world it can be very easy to identify who we are or are not biologically related to.

> I'm a scientist, I know how easy it is these days for kids to do a few basic tests and find out that their parents might not be their biological parents. So really, it's logical. It's stupid to put it off because it's even nastier for them to discover it by themselves. (Carl)

> It's his right to know. When he gets older he's going to have to know. If he had an accident, he might say, 'Why can't you give me blood Dad?' It's only fair to him. (Paul)

Past experiences in families can affect many things we do. Pam, like Patrice and I, made her initial decision about telling her son based on family events.

> We never intended to lie, mainly because of the experience of my cousin who was quite devastated to find out, at the age of forty, that she was adopted. Everyone in her family knew except her and she felt terribly deceived. She was relieved also, she knew there was something different about her but she didn't know what. So, we knew we were going to tell our child at some point.

As we have already said, keeping a secret can be a huge emotional load. It is a burden that some parents do not want to carry, as Chris describes.

We thought we were going to maintain the 'family secret' of our child's conception, he would never find out, so he would never have any concerns of being created in this different manner.

We both decided to tell our son when we had our second child, he was six years old, and we had both been feeling increasingly uncomfortable with basing our family relationships around a secret. A lie, call it what you want, it just felt so wrong and was beginning to cause friction for us as a couple, trying to keep this 'family secret.' A lot of energy goes into maintaining a secret, especially one so important as this, and believe me it is such wasted energy. It felt a lot like sitting on a time bomb, waiting for it to go off. Our son was becoming an individual and becoming aware of his family and relatives that lived overseas and the wider community in general. He had been with me on many occasions visiting the clinic for ultrasounds and injections, with the IVF cycle that produced his sister, so this in itself made him aware that his parents needed help to have babies.

Many like Chris feel that they need honesty within their families in order to function properly. Belinda is a firm believer in this.

I have always been a strong advocate for complete honesty, especially in important relationships. I don't see how you can possibly have a close and strong relationship with a child that you have lied to about something as fundamental as their conception and genetics. Michael's biggest concern has always been whether the child will truly look on him as their father. It seems that all the children who are told about their conception early have had good relationships with their dad, but those who were lied to, and most likely found out later, didn't. That just seems logical to me, because children are very perceptive, and if you're hiding something like that, they would know that something's not quite right, so how could they feel safe? Apart from anything else, donor conception is nothing to be ashamed of and if we tried to hide it, it would be as though there was something to hide.

Of course, there are still parents who feel that the right thing to do is to keep the method of a child's conception from them. I have never spoken to a parent who was 100 percent sure about keeping the truth of donor conception from their child. Even those who said they would not tell their child still left the door open a tiny bit.

We live in a country area and we have decided not to tell our children. I think our children could be treated differently if people knew. I don't think our parents would look on our children the same way. That's not to say that one day we might not change our minds, maybe after our parents are gone. (Lori)

Will I tell the child? I don't know. I'm scared to and scared not to. We are not sure that openness would be best for us. Our families are not open to many new things. They were critical about infertility treatment to begin with. We aren't sure we want the complications that telling everyone might bring. We have decided to wait and see how things turn out, who knows we might decide to tell. The father is the man who is raising the child, not the one giving the sperm. (Lisa)

Uncertainty can divide families where one parent would like to tell and the other feels the need to keep things secret or where no concrete decisions about telling have been made. This is what Julie's husband wanted.

The question as to whether or not to tell my children about their origin never came up. My husband wanted nothing to do with telling the children or even thinking about how they were conceived. (Julie)

Julie went ahead and told her children how they were conceived.

To this day, he has never spoken a word to either child about their biological background. Neither the children nor I have ever asked him why he hasn't wanted to discuss the issue. The entire subject has been left to me. I grew up in a family where many actual lies were told to me and many underlying secrets swam around in the family. I knew for sure my children were going to live in a family where everything was truthful and above board.

Counseling before embarking on a donor conception program is essential for prospective recipient parents. It will give them the opportunity to work through issues to do with telling children. Parents-to-be must come to a decision about this vital issue before conceiving their child. If parents cannot agree, then perhaps donor conception is not for them.

I honestly believe that the vast majority of parents do want to tell their children but the numbers who actually do, even though they are growing, are still limited. Lack of support services may account for the small numbers of parents telling; families are living with a secret they do not necessarily support. Within the area of adoption, most countries have government or religious organizations that facilitate the adoption process. These organizations usually also provide long-term support for adoptive families and this support includes talking to children about their adoption. Nothing like this exists for donor-conceived families. While counselors at some infertility clinics can help, many do not have experience in the area of genetic origin information, so volunteer support groups like the DCSG and DC Network are for many the only avenues of advice and support. The next two chapters will give help to families in this area by sharing the experiences of parents who have told their children.

9

Telling Our Children

What do families do if they want to tell their children? As we discussed in the last chapter, there is very little in the way of formal support for parents who want to tell their children the truth of their conception. So, the best answers at the moment would be to read books like this and learn as much as possible about the subject. Seek out support groups which are a great way of meeting with other parents of donor-conceived children. Learn as much as you can about how they told their children, how they coped with any questions their children asked. Also, recipient parents should go back to the clinic they attended and speak to the counselor, ask their advice. Or even talk to a family counselor or psychologist. Doing one or all of these things will not result in the perfect way to tell a child about donor conception, but it will give a number of examples and ideas that can be thought about. Then parents should be in a better position to come up with a way they think will suit their individual situation and family.

Jenny had originally been advised by her doctor to never tell her children about their conception by donated gametes but after a number of years she felt that this was not right for her family. She consulted a psychiatrist who suggested that they should be told as early as possible.

> We were advised by a psychiatrist the earlier the better, so both Kylie and Glenn were told at seven years old. I remember Kylie's reply was to ask if we could go to the Melbourne Cup. I was so taken aback after trying to explain this delicate subject, and I thought, 'I didn't do very well at that, she didn't understand a thing I said.' So we talked some more and she'd taken in all she could for a seven year old – it was just no big deal. Whenever the chance comes up now I speak about DI and they accept it as part of their life. (And no, we still haven't been to a Melbourne Cup.)

Evelyn and Laurie were also told by their doctor never to tell their two children. When they did decide to tell they, like Jenny, consulted a professional. Their children, who are now in their late twenties, were near the end of their primary schooling when they were told.

> We worried about what the repercussions of telling might be. (Evelyn)

> I worried about rejection. I probably shouldn't have, there was no reason to worry. (Laurie)

> We sat them down, we planned it very carefully, we had several appointments with a psychologist, as a couple together and one each separately. We thought by going to a psychologist that if the children did take it badly then we would have professional back-up so not too much damage would be done to them. We devised a little play act on how to tell them, what we would say. We rehearsed our words, chose them very carefully, we didn't want them to misinterpret what we were really wanting to say. We carefully planned the time that we thought would be a good time to tell them. We chose the time just before Nigel went to high school; we knew that we would have to tell him before he had all the pressures of high school and puberty. We were told by the psychologist not to take them out somewhere to tell them because they'd have nowhere to go if they felt badly about it, they couldn't go off and brood. She said tell them one night and take them out for a little celebration the next night.
> We were lucky with what was going on with IVF babies at the time. We would deliberately sit them down in front of the news and say, 'Look at these little babies, oh they're just so loved and so wanted, they're special babies.' So, along the way we were sort of preparing them. That was what we focussed on, that they were desperately wanted children.
> When we sat them down that night we said, 'We've got something special to tell you' and Nigel said, 'I know, I was adopted wasn't I?'
> We didn't think that they understood what we were saying because after we told them Nigel saw his mate out the front playing football and said, 'Oh, there's Nathan, I'm going out to play football with him.' They both went outside without saying a word. We looked at one another and said, 'Well, I really don't know whether they understood what we were talking about.' There was no reaction, there were no questions, no anything.
> We told them on the Saturday and on the Sunday night when I came home from work I said, 'Right kids, it's your choice, we're going to go out and have a little celebration about our special family.' It was right on

Christmas, just after Nigel's birthday, and he knew that finances were a bit tight. He said, 'We don't have to go out to dinner.' He put his arm around his father and said, 'Nothing's been changed, Dad's my dad and he always will be.' The tears were there, we knew that he understood exactly what he'd been told. (Evelyn)

Evelyn and Laurie had spent time planning how to tell their children in the best way they knew how. Gwen and Paul had also planned a special time in which to tell their two daughters, as Gwen relates.

The oldest one was fourteen, the other one must have been just under ten. We'd been trying to tell them for about two years, planning a day. I always chickened out. It wasn't any big deal in the end. The only reason I did panic was because Paul was afraid that 'we might stuff it up.' I felt that if we did I would have to take all the blame because I was more eager to tell them.

On the night we told them we bought tea and made everything comfy at home and left the telly on so we didn't have to make a real big deal about it; you know if you turn the telly off there's something definitely wrong I talked about donating blood, stuff like that. The youngest one is very medically minded, quite smart, and I thought it would really interest her. I said, 'You know how lots of babies are born by IVF?' (Paul's cousin has got twins that are IVF and I mentioned them.) I talked about how babies can be born differently or made differently. I used simple language. They said, 'What, are we adopted?' so I just had to blurt it out because they were panicking thinking they were adopted. They sighed with relief. They didn't fully understand what it was about, which was what I expected, but they didn't have any questions either.

The next day the oldest one came and asked, 'Does that mean Nana isn't really our Nana?' and I said, 'Oh well, I guess it really does.' You can't lie to them. I said, 'All Daddy's side aren't biologically related.' I think for a while they felt that they didn't really belong anywhere because most of my family have departed.

The next day they made up a little card on the computer, with, 'Thank you, we love you both,' all that sort of stuff. It was so touching, it was so thoughtful. When I told them, I said that it was best to be honest with them and I think they appreciate that. I think they've grown up to really appreciate what that meant for us, how hard it was.

I told them honestly that the reason we hadn't told them earlier was that we just didn't know how to. We didn't have any support (about telling) and I had thought, 'God, if they go off the rails, there's no one there to back us up.' There wasn't even a Nan there to say, 'Look love, Mum tried to do her best.' Adoption is different, maybe easier, because in adoption they know there are other kids out there who were adopted, but they don't know with this. Look at half the adults you talk to, they don't know about DI.

I thought my oldest child would tell friends. She's grown up with one girl almost since they were born. I found out about a year later that she'd told her practically the next day. We didn't tell them they couldn't tell anyone else. We said that some day they might feel like telling someone but that you don't want to tell everybody. I don't think the youngest one has told anyone. I told some girlfriends last year, but before that I hadn't told anyone. Paul's really more open now, he's more confident about himself. It's healthy; it's so much better.

Leonie and Warren wanted their eldest daughter to know that children come into families in many different ways.

We wrote our words down and we role-played it. (Leonie)

We wanted to do it in a loving environment to let her know that it was something really special. We wanted to make her feel good about the experience and to let her know that it wasn't something that we were ashamed of. We both were worried about her reaction. I think the biggest fear is rejection, you think they might jump up and say, 'You're not my father, not really my father.' It was really all in my own mind. (Warren)

On the night we told her we took the phone off the hook and got take-away tea. We sat her down and said, 'We've got something to tell you tonight. We want to tell you how babies are born, how they come into the world and that some people can't have babies because their bodies don't work well. You know that Matthew [a friend down the street] is adopted? When his parents first got married their bodies didn't work well for them and they really wanted a family. Matthew needed a family to go to, and they adopted him, and that's how he came to be in their family. You know there is another way that people come into families, sometimes the man can't make the sperm that helps to make a baby, or a woman's body doesn't work properly. If a man is having problems with his sperm you can go to a hospital and a kind man gives his sperm to help people like us have children.' At the end of it she said, 'We should buy that man a present.' We said, 'There is really no need to buy that man a gift because he has given us the greatest gift of all.'

> She was told that there were lots of children born this way, that she could talk to us about it at any time. We explained that she couldn't tell her friends because their parents would like to tell their own children the way babies are born. The following day we told her school-teacher, because we wanted the teacher to know about it if Geraldine said things at school. Her teacher said, 'Yes, Geraldine did say one day that Mum and Dad are trying to have another baby.' (Leonie)

This careful planning and thought made them feel a bit more confident when they came to tell their other two children.

> It was a lot easier telling the other two. I think it was a little bit different telling a boy because you have a different sort of a relationship with a boy. Boys like to be like their dads. I guess there was a little bit of apprehension there as well because all kids are different. When we told Keiron he was never really interested in babies, he was more interested in how you got the sperm out. He was told during the school holidays because we wanted him to have two weeks at home, so that if he had any questions he could talk about them with us and not have to go and deal with it at school. Kieron asked things like: 'How does the sperm get out, do you just press a button?', 'Is it the same man for Geraldine and Genevieve?' We said, 'No, it's three different men.' We didn't explain about the fact that there might be half-siblings to them, but Geraldine knows now. (Warren)

Even with planning, things don't always work out the way we expect. Parents can have questions sprung on them when they least expect it. Becky had not yet told her children about how they were conceived when her eldest son suddenly asked her about where babies come from.

> It happened when I wasn't prepared for it. My eldest son came home from school confused. His friend had told him (kindergarten class) that babies came from eggs. We had just incubated duck eggs and he thought that strange. I explained about egg and sperm and got out a book called *Where did I come from?* I was divorced, and I suppose due to the divorce Brandon asked me point blank if the sperm that made him came from my ex-husband.

The moment of truth was in my face and I wasn't ready. I didn't want to lie, however, so I told him no, that a special man helped us as Bill didn't have good sperm. I think Brandon was six at the time. The twins listened in, but I don't think anything really 'registered.' If you ask them when they were told, they will look to me for the answer, because they don't know. They have always known, as far as they are concerned. It is also no big deal to them.

When our eldest son, Andrew, was two years old Patrice and I decided to try to have another child. Andrew was a very curious child and we knew that coming with me to the hospital when I had blood tests would inevitably arouse his curiosity. Before our first visit to the clinic we sat him down and explained things as simply as possible.

To create a baby you need a sperm from the daddy and an egg from the mummy. In our family Daddy doesn't have any sperm, so to be able to have you we had to go to a clinic. At the clinic, the doctor got some sperm from a man who wanted to help people like us to have babies. Now we want to have another baby, so we have to go to the clinic at the hospital to get some more sperm. Mummy has to have blood taken from her for a few days so the clinic will know the right time to give us the sperm.

At the time, this explanation elicited no questions from Andrew. When we got to the clinic, he was fascinated by the blood coming out of my arm and was fussed over by the nurses who would give him disposable tweezers and other instruments to play with.

To tell a child about their creation by donor conception when they are very young – under five years of age – is not an extremely difficult thing to do. Some parents start telling their children when they are still babes in arms. By doing this, parents have plenty of time to listen to themselves speak the words about donor conception. When their children are old enough to need more explanations, or when they ask questions, the parents will feel quite comfortable about what they are saying and the vocabulary they are using.

Vivianne and Michael decided that this would be the best way for their family.

When I was breastfeeding her I'd just talk about the way she was born, and eventually I reached a point where she started to connect and ask me questions. When she got older I'd say, 'I think you've got your donor's colour hair,' things like that. We explained to her the process. Daddy didn't have any sperm and that women have eggs. Mummy had to get sperm from the hospital from another man called the donor.

She got upset once when she asked whether her cousins and friends had been born the same way as her and I had said, 'No, their daddies had sperm.' She got very upset, felt she was different, so what I did was tell her that she was 'born' the same way as her cousins – her aunty, friend's mothers and me all had our own eggs and that she and they were all born the same way. She liked that; she felt that connected her.

Now, after that incident, when I approach the subject it's more on the connection side so she feels she belongs and is not apart. She knows her daddy doesn't have sperm, she totally understands that. She talked to Elizabeth [a friend of the same age also born by DI] about it at the last support group picnic. She said, 'You were born the same way as me, your daddy didn't have any sperm, just like mine.'

Other parents wait until their children are a little older, as Patrice and I did. Janet and Julian took an opportunity that arose on their farm to tell their son.

We started telling when Oscar was three. He's a very lively, curious, clever little fellow and one day when we were artificially inseminating the dairy cows Oscar wanted to know what we were doing. We said, 'These are the seeds from the bull and they go into the cow's egg.' Then we explained that it could be that way with people, too, that there are lots of different ways of making families.

Later at home we sat down with the book *My Story* and explained in very simple terms that we had wanted to have a baby desperately but it wasn't happening. We went and had some tests and the doctor said that Daddy didn't have any seeds. We went to a hospital where they had seeds from lots of different men, and we picked one, and that went with Mummy's eggs and made this fantastic boy, Oscar. He just accepted it like any other story we had read. He asked, 'Can we get more seeds, can we have more babies?' We replied that we were not sure about that. He asked, 'Who is he?' We said, 'A nice man who did this for us.' Oscar also asked questions about how they put the seeds with the egg, and where and how the baby grows.

I've heard Oscar tell friends about it already. He'll just kind of say something about seeds and people react by pretending they don't hear. He's very open and I dare say that if a classroom discussion starts on things Oscar will introduce the idea, and for that reason I have told his teacher about it. It's a difficult thing because you don't want to perpetuate this whole secrecy thing but at the same time you don't want your child getting hurt.

Joanne also told her eldest child at quite a young age as she felt that Lauran would be able to understand the information about her conception.

Lauran remembers coming to the clinic with me when Ian was conceived. I started talking to her very early, on our seven-hour trips in the car to the clinic. You could have a conversation with Lauran when she was eighteen months old; we used to call her Granny. From that time she knew, but the big push came when she was five and a half; there was something on TV about DI and they were advertising the book *Where did I Come From? The story of donor insemination*. I rang my sister who lived in Sydney and she got it for me. We read the book to Lauran and Ian, and then we said, 'Daddy's sperm is dead,' and Lauran said, 'Well I'm glad Daddy's sperm's dead and not Daddy.' That's the way she dealt with it.

Rob told his son when Jack was about three years old.

When Jack could understand we told him he was a very special child. We told him that Daddy didn't have any sperm and a kind man at the hospital donated sperm to us. That was enough to satisfy his interest. I can remember one day driving Jack back from kindergarten. He was sitting in the back of the car and out of the blue he said, 'I've got a good idea Daddy, if you haven't got any sperm then you can have some of mine,' which I thought was a sweet, childlike understanding of the situation.

Julie, like thousands of other recipient parents, had no idea when she should tell her children, so she decided that the earlier the better.

For some reason I thought that when each child was eighteen months old I should tell them, 'Daddy is their daddy, but he did not make them.' I'm sure they had no concept of what I was talking about or why I would say such a thing. They took the information, added it to their minds, and continued to develop in a healthy fashion. Because I had little information as to when the correct time was to tell my children, I decided to err on the too early side, versus too late. By too late, I mean after an incident happens that the biological background is brought out without the child knowing beforehand.

I think it is so important for them to know, especially when it comes to genetics. Our doctor, who forgot about their biological background, asked my daughter if her father wore glasses. My daughter relayed to me her answer 'I told her I didn't know, and she looked at me real funny.' My daughter and I both kind of giggled at the weirdness of the situation.

Anne and Carl's daughter, Amy, is still very young, but they have spent time planning how they will tell her about her conception by donor egg and what words they will use.

We're very open about donor eggs in front of our daughter, from the day she came home we've talked about it. She doesn't understand anything of it yet, but there's that air of openness. I write a letter to our donor every year, they haven't been passed on because my husband doesn't want that yet.

I haven't gone into a great deal of depth with my daughter about her conception, as she's only eighteen months old. I have a plan for a book that I will put together for her. The sorts of things I plan to put in her book are things like 'Once upon a time there was a little girl called Amy and she lived with her mum and dad, Carl and Anne. They used to be very unhappy. They wanted to have a baby but they couldn't. All babies grow from an egg and a sperm and so did Amy. Carl had sperm to make a baby but Anne didn't have any eggs.

'Anne's doctor asked a kind woman if she would share some of her eggs with them. She said yes. Carl and Anne were very excited. At last, they might be able to have a baby of their own.

'The doctor put some of Carl's sperm with the woman's eggs. Some of the eggs and sperm joined together and started to grow into embryos. The doctor put the embryos inside Anne. Everyone hoped that the embryos would keep growing.

'One embryo did keep growing into a baby. Anne and Carl were so happy. The baby kept growing inside her mum until she was ready to be born. When she was born, her mum and dad were very happy. They loved her very, very much and called her Amy.'

Single women and lesbian couples choose to create a child who will have no father present from birth. Children can sometimes notice differences in their families from a very young age; they may ask questions quite early on about why there are fathers in other families but none in theirs. Most mothers I have spoken to who have no male partner have chosen to tell their donor-conceived child about his or her conception at a very young age, as Karen did.

> I began to write a book for him before he was born. It begins with my decision to have him and follows my pregnancy, his birth, and continues on. It actually has turned into a yearbook and I give him a new chapter each Christmas as his life unfolds. I read it with him. He mainly likes to talk about the pictures of him, his family, and friends. He knows that he and I are a family and that his grandparents and his cousins, uncles and aunts are part of his 'bigger' family.
>
> I hope he grows up feeling very full and satisfied with his life. I do hope that I will not remain single and that some day there will be a special man in our lives that he will grow to love and call 'Daddy.' If this doesn't happen, I hope he will be happy with the ties he has with his uncles and my male friends. My biggest fear is that he will not feel complete without knowing his biological father. I think that the system of not offering DI offspring this opportunity robs many of the children of a full life! I hope there is a change to regulations and that my son will be able to access any answers he may need.

The reasons many parents don't tell their children until they are older are extremely varied. Some feel that there is no point because the child will have no comprehension of conception and birth at a very young age. Others will explain about birth but will add the particulars about donor conception when they feel the child will understand. Some will wait until their child asks questions about where babies come from. Of course, there will always be some children who ask no questions about this until they are leaving childhood, and others ask none at all, preferring to gain their knowledge from friends.

A great number of parents I have spoken to have postponed telling their children because they have no idea how to do it. This can sometimes result in the telling being put off and put off until they feel they can delay no longer. Vivianne had wanted to tell her children for quite some time but had been unsure how to go about it. After talking to someone at a support group, she finally decided that the time had come.

> My children were seven-and-a-half when I told them. I let them know that babies come into the world in all different ways, that they are very special to me and Daddy, and that they were really wanted. My body wasn't working properly at the time so this nice kind lady helped me out

by sharing her eggs with me. I remember my son saying, 'Oh, I don't get it, shouldn't we be with her?' I said, 'No, I'll explain to you how eggs are taken from the body and how other people can use them.' My son asked, 'What did she look like?' I said, 'Well, I'm not sure, but she must have been lovely looking because look at you two.' My daughter asked, 'What was her name?' and I replied, 'I don't know, but we can find a name for her,' and my daughter said, 'Let's call her Belinda.' I was so nervous about telling them and felt my stomach was in knots. After I told them they went straight to sleep, very secure, snoring happily, while I was in the bathroom with a bout of gastric but feeling relieved for at last having told them the truth.

The other day my daughter asked me, 'What is the thing that gives the colour of your eyes and hair?' I replied, 'They're called genes.' I didn't want to go into it in any great length but I tried to explain what genes were. I told them that they've got the genes of Daddy and the genes of the lady that helped me, but they have my blood running through their veins because they grew in my tummy. Referring to the 'lady that helped us out' my daughter said very confidently, with a smile on her face, 'Oh yes, it's almost like she's our ex-mother.' I thought, that's clever, I hadn't thought of that.

Like Vivianne, Pam and David also felt more sure of themselves after talking to other parents.

Lachlan was five when we went to a seminar on telling your children about donor conception. That really gave us the confidence to do something. We waited for the right moment, and when something came up on TV about six babies born from some fertility treatment we took it up from there. Really it was easy. We said that there's this other man that helped us and that we had to go to the hospital. I think we might have used the word 'seed' initially but we've now changed that to 'sperm'. We read the book *My Story* to him but he didn't really seem that interested. A couple of nights later we got the same book out again to try and reinforce it, but he said, 'We've read that one, I want another one.' We bring it up now and then but we haven't tried to push it, we'll just wait for him to come to a point where he wants to know a bit more.

Like Pam and David, there are many parents, especially those telling quite young children, who feel better if they have something with which to help explain things. A number have used books such as *My Story*, which is specifically designed to explain DI to young children. Irene and her husband, Peter, used these same books to aid in their explanations, and planned very carefully how they would expand the story as their children grew.

> We've read a couple of books to the kids *My Story* and *Mommy Did I grow in Your Tummy?* to the kids on and off but there wasn't really a lot of interest at the time with the kids being quite young. We felt we would start off simple and let them take the lead. Sharing this with the kids has led us to have talks about the baby in Mommy's 'tummy' (we tried uterus, but tummy won out with the kids for now) and how an egg from a woman and sperm from a man can make a baby.
>
> We would add in bits of our story about not being able to make a baby together, being very sad about this, and going to the doctor to try to make a baby. We mentioned that we were able to use the sperm from a man who gave it to the doctor so that people like their mommy and Daddy could make a baby. We mentioned how happy we were that this man did this and that our wonderful children were here with us now. They never commented on this at the time.

Karen, who was divorced, wanted to be alone with her son when she told him. She is another parent who used a book to aid in telling her son.

> It was just Brad and I, we went down to the beach for the day, got a secluded spot and we had a picnic. We played for an hour and then I just said, 'Well, now you're ten it's time to tell you the facts of life.' A few questions had come up about that anyway. He got all giggly and stupid. I covered up the donor insemination words on the front of the book, *My Story* and then I said, 'This is how people began but you are actually special, you were born by donor insemination.' We read the book and I thought I would break down and cry, but I didn't. He said, 'I had no idea.' Brad actually looks like his dad. I explained how DI worked because I didn't want him to think that I'd been off with another man. He fully understood it all. He was very grown up about it.

Of course, the amount and type of questions that a child might ask on being told about their conception by donated gametes will depend on a variety of things, including their age, their interest in the subject, and their understanding of it. A great many, on being told, will ask few or no questions at all. Some will even appear to have no interest in the subject. We should never take this to mean that they are not thinking about things.

If a child asks no questions I think it is good to reassure them that if they ever do want to ask something they should feel free to do so. With our own children, Patrice and I have taken opportunities such as news stories about infertility to bring up the topic of donor conception again. Then we can either go over the story or add further information, and this gives them the opportunity to ask us questions. There is more about this in the next chapter.

So far we have talked about infertile parents, or mothers without male partners, telling their children, but what about people like John who used DI for genetic reasons? Will he tell his children any differently?

> We actually decided that prior to going through with this we would tell them at some stage. The exact time for that we haven't decided yet. My feeling is probably when our youngest child, Matthew, is old enough to understand, then we'll tell them both together. I believe it will be easy to explain to them as long as they understand how a baby is conceived. My daughter has noticed things for some time because I have quite a deal of scarring on my elbows, knees, hands and feet which is very visible, it looks like I've had a bad burn. I have no fingernails and no toenails, and that's very noticeable for a child. She has asked things like 'Daddy why haven't you got fingernails?', 'Daddy have you hurt yourself?', 'Daddy you've got a Band-Aid on.' At this stage we just say that Daddy's got a bit of a problem, and later on I think it will be easier to explain things to her. We will explain that we didn't want to use Daddy's sperm because they would probably have been born with the same problem.
>
> I think from my perspective it should be easy for them to accept. That's probably very naïve; I suppose we'll just have to cross that bridge when we come to it. I think children are just so much more intelligent on these things nowadays. They can't avoid hearing things on the TV about test-tube babies, and so on. I don't think that the expressions and the terminology we're going to use when we're talking about DI will be all that foreign to them by the time we get around to it.

As I have said, because of the lack of information and advice on how to tell their children about donor conception parents can tie themselves up in knots about how to do it. They can put it off, sometimes for years, and some even decide they cannot do it at all.

Richard tells how he felt after agonizing over whether to tell his child about her conception using donor sperm and then finally telling her.

> What a weight I feel lifted off me now there are no more secrets. We can build on trust now that all the cards are on the table.

10

After the Telling

After parents have told their donor-conceived children about the way in which they came into the world, what do they do next? Is the subject forgotten, or is it a regular topic of conversation? Will these children have a huge amount of curiosity about the subject and their donor? Will the subject affect them deeply? Or will the opposite be true, and will they have no interest at all?

I don't think there is anyway that this sort of information can ever not affect someone. It is only natural that children will have questions and be curious about the method of their conception and about their donor.

When telling children about their conception using donated gametes, I feel we must be sure to never tell them once and then put the subject away. In very young children, an occasional repeat of the story is helpful so that they don't forget it and also to add to their understanding as they grow. But one of the most important reasons for parents to raise the topic again is to let their children know that the subject is always open for discussion and that they welcome any questions about it. There can be nothing worse than a child desperately wanting to ask questions and being afraid to. Stories about reproductive technology often appear in the media, and this can be a starter for discussions about donor conception. For young children, pregnant friends or relatives can also allow an easy entry into the subject of donor conception.

Olivia's children have grown up with the knowledge of their conception and she reinforces the idea I have mentioned of repeating the topic of donor conception with children over time.

We started the process of telling when our eldest was about four-and-a-half, using a *How Babies are Made* picture book and adapting it. We also took opportunities to mention differences in ways babies are made when friends had babies. The youngest has just grown up with DI 'being around.' Neither can remember a time when they didn't know. William, the eldest, asked lots of questions following reading *My Story*. He has asked virtually nothing since (he's now sixteen and a half), except if we knew if his donor is bald (he doesn't want to go bald early)! He told me recently, on being questioned, that he has no curiosity about his donor (probably not true, but he is a very private person). His sister, on the other hand, has always been very open, asks questions, talks to her friends, and is curious about her donor.

Olivia brings up a very important point. While children may say to their parents that they have no curiosity about the donor it might not be the way they truly feel. Probably a great many offspring worry about how their curiosity might affect their parents. This makes it even more important to keep lines of communication open and bring up the topic occasionally so that children know that the subject of donor conception is open to questions and discussion.

As mentioned in the previous chapter, books can be useful to parents when they first tell their children but can be useful also in consolidating that information over time. Irene and Peter have a selection of books for children on reproductive technology.

Our DI books are in the 'mud room,' which is basically where our home office is, and one to two weeks ago Megan pulled out the books and asked me to read them to her. Adam was playing. He sat down after a bit and asked if it was OK if I started again from the beginning.

While I was reading the part about the sperm donors and mentioned again that was how Mommy and Daddy were able to have them, Adam asked me if I had a picture of our donor. I told him no, we didn't, and we didn't know very much about him. I asked Adam why he wanted a picture of him, and he said he just wanted to know what he looked like. I finished reading the books and then thought, OK, I'll try to take this one step further and see where it leads us.

I asked them both what would they say if they could say something to their donor? Adam piped up that he would ask him if he could draw a picture of himself. I asked him why, and he said he wanted to know what he looked like and to make sure he wasn't a vampire or something like that. Adam has quite an imagination and at around that time was talking about vampires. Then Megan said in her sweet little voice, with her eye-lashes fluttering, 'I'd tell him that I love him.' When I asked her why, she said that she loved him because he helped us make a baby and she loved babies.

And where was Peter during all of this? He was working on the computer and came out shortly afterwards. I told him that we read the stories and about my question to the kids, and asked him to ask the kids himself. They basically told him what they had said. We both thought it went very well, considering it was our first 'conversation,' and that was the end of talking about DI or donors that night.

Some time later Irene wrote more about talking to her children.

Amy is being baptized this coming Sunday and I was explaining to Megan and Adam how baptism is a special ceremony where baby Amy will be welcomed into God's family. Then we talked a bit about their baptisms, and I said I'd show them their pictures of their own baptisms later. After a few minutes Adam, out of the blue remarked, 'When Daddy's sperm couldn't make a baby, we used the sperm from another man's 'collection' and the doctor put it inside your tummy and it made a baby.' I said yes, that's how we were able to have all of you! I chuckled to myself at his choice of the word 'collection' (he's into collecting stuff right now) and thought to myself, this is sinking in.

As my mind is wandering, I'm thinking 'I wonder how this would go over if he mentions this to his playschool class.' With Peter or myself not being there to support him and explain, it could be most interesting, or disastrous! So perhaps now is the time to mention that this is our 'special' family story and we usually only talk about it with our family. I don't want him to think there is something wrong, but perhaps this is a time to plant the seed of privacy. Or would that just encourage the opposite?

Lately our daughter, Megan, has been asking more questions about their donor, and she's really curious about babies. She plays with her dolls, sticks them under her shirt, and says she's going to have one. She wants to be a mommy and have babies when she's grown up. She pretends to breastfeed her dolls (I'm still nursing our youngest) and has been wanting to read the DI books more so than her older brother.

The other day she absolutely floored me when I was reading *My Story*. We were at the page with the picture of the three donors sitting on chairs and she asked me, 'Mommy, I have a question…why do the sperm donors give away their sperm to make a baby? Don't they want to keep it to make children with their own wives if they have them?' This is from a four-year-old! So we talked about how some donors may not have families and their own children yet, but that they want to help other mommies and daddies like us have children. And then she says, 'And make their dreams come true!' She must have remembered this comment from one of her books, or Disney tapes…She's a very mature four-year-old at times.

A few weeks ago Megan and Adam were playing doctor and I went in to check on them. My daughter's bunny was lying on the bed, and she pronounced that the bunny was going to have a baby and held up a plastic toy egg and a beaded necklace which she called the sperm from the donor, and so on they played. I don't know if this type of play happens in preschool…but I don't think so at this point. And I'm really not worried. I guess we'll cross that bridge when we get to it.

We're talking about privacy issues with the kids now, too. Keeping their private body parts covered except from their parents, or doctors if they are having a check up. You don't go running around showing them to everyone, and we hope to talk a bit about private family information and use their DI origins as an example. I'm not sure how that will go, but I don't want to give them the impression that to talk about DI is negative, just that it's not something we talk about to everyone.

As Irene and Peter have found the questions or comments from younger children can be quite touching or humorous, and other parents have found the same thing.

> Genevieve said to Warren one time, 'I think that the men and ladies who can't have babies are nicer,' and another time, 'It doesn't matter that Dad doesn't have healthy sperm it just matters that he loves and enjoys children a lot.' (Leonie)

Evelyn and Laurie have also had their lighter moments.

> I always tell the story about one night when I was peeling the vegetables and my two children had a ding-dong of a barny. Lauren came out to me and Nigel had been giving her a real bad time and she said, 'Mum, Nigel's donor must be an awful man.' I asked, 'What makes you think that?' and she said, 'Because he's nothing like you.' After that we did joke about the donor and he'd cop any of the negative traits. (Evelyn)

That was lucky because I didn't! (Laurie)

Bad habits, they were blamed on genetics, blamed on the donor. We've always said that telling our children made our relationship stronger. It was a heavy load lifted off our shoulders, the burden that we'd been carrying for all those years was gone, we didn't have any secrets from them any longer. I think they realized over the years how painful it must have been on us, especially when they know there are people out there who aren't telling their children at all. That's one passion Nigel does have, that children should be told. I don't think that the relationship between Nigel and Lauren and Laurie could be any stronger even if they were biologically connected. Nigel went away fishing with Laurie for the whole week up the river not long ago. Nigel always used to come home from school in the teenage years and say about his mate, 'He hates his parents.' He could never get over this best mate hating his parents. You always knew that the love was there. (Evelyn)

Evelyn and Laurie have worked to bring about laws regarding donor conception in their home state of Victoria, they want all donor offspring to be able to know who their donors are when they become adults. Evelyn and Laurie are in a unique position to give us an insight into how siblings in one family can feel differently about information on their donors. While their eldest child, Nigel, has no interest in his donor, Lauren really wanted to have information about him.

Nigel's a firm believer that children should be told. I think that he thinks that we're thumping our head against a brick wall (trying to bring in laws), but he realizes that we're making it better for future children even though he says that, 'It's not going to alter anything for Lauren and me.' We don't know how he's going to react when he has a child of his own, what feelings it will bring out in him, maybe it doesn't hit them until they have their own children. (Evelyn)

Lauren and her parents tried to get donor information for Lauren but were told it no longer exists.

If Lauren knew that her donor's information was there she probably would want to have it, but she's not letting it consume her or rule her life at this stage. (Evelyn)

We started telling our eldest son when he was about two years old as I described in the previous chapter. When our other two children were born they were never 'sat down and told,' it was more a matter of their being around when we were talking about DI with Andrew, and if they weren't then we would do a rerun of the conversation at the dinner table. This was also a good way for my husband to get to hear what the children were thinking and to join in the discussion. As many mothers know, they are often the ones that most questions are aimed at – mainly because they tend to be the ones at home with the young children during the day.

Callum, our second son, now eight, never asked any questions about DI when he was very young, he never appeared to be even remotely interested. When he was six he asked me how people got to be people. I thought that he was asking about how babies were born but he said no, that he wanted to know how the people got out of the sea! He meant that he wanted to know about evolution, so we had a brief discussion about it and then he asked about how babies start growing in their 'Mummy's tummies.' I told him how the sperm gets into the egg and it starts to grow cells to make a baby. He thought that the egg must have a 'hatch' in it so that the sperm could get in. He asked about how twins and triplets came to be, and we talked briefly about that. I took the opportunity to talk to him about donor insemination.

I said, 'You know how you need an egg from the mum and a sperm from the dad to make a baby?' He nodded. 'Well, in our family we had a problem, Daddy didn't have any sperm.' His immediate response was, 'I knew that!' I asked him if he knew where we got the sperm from, he replied, 'Yes, from a stranger!'

I suggested that perhaps 'stranger' wasn't quite the right word for the man who gave us the sperm. I didn't want him to confuse it with 'stranger danger' – but, on second thoughts I think he knew that the proper meaning of 'stranger' is someone we don't know. I went on to talk with him about how the man gave his sperm to the hospital to help people like us who couldn't have a baby, and that the hospital gave it to us. That was the end of our conversation as he had obviously had enough of it and went off to play.

So Callum had been absorbing the information all along and so far has never felt the need to ask questions, but at least now we have had a little talk about donor conception and he knows he can ask us about it in future.

Callum's older brother, Andrew, seems to have a bit more curiosity about his conception and has asked questions. When he was nearly seven he read a front-page newspaper article about IVF twins. They had been conceived with sperm from two different men because there had been a mix-up with phials of sperm. There were quite a few things about the article that Andrew didn't understand, and while I was explaining them we talked about donor sperm. We talked about why Daddy didn't have any sperm. I also told Andrew that when we go to Donor Conception Support Group barbeques that most of the dads there don't have any of their own sperm to make a baby and that the other children there were made the same way he was. Then Andrew asked a very thoughtful question: 'But why do we need a support group?' It took me a second to try to think of a way to explain that he might understand. I said that many husbands and wives get very sad that they can't have a baby that comes from both of their bodies. I added that many people find it hard to explain to their children about how they were conceived by sperm that was given by another man. Going to support group meetings helped us by giving us the chance to talk over things with other parents just like us.

Andrew then asked if I would like to meet the man who gave us the sperm (I'd already explained to him that we didn't know who the donor was). I answered that we probably would never be able to meet him as the clinic kept it a secret, but that one day, if he wanted to, we could find out something about the donor. Andrew then asked the one question that I couldn't answer in a way that he could understand. 'Why is it a secret?' After that Andrew didn't seem interested in the discussion any more and went off to play. He hadn't seemed worried at all that I couldn't answer his last question properly.

When he was about eight we were in the supermarket fruit and veg section. I was picking out tomatoes and Andrew was across the other side of the aisle, looking at all the varieties of nuts. He said in a loud voice, 'I think I'm so bright because of the man who gave us the sperm.' Well, what do you say to a statement like that? 'Maybe you're right,' I said. 'Did Dad have enough sperm for Callum?' 'No,' I answered. 'Did he have enough for Elizabeth?' 'No.'

The conversation ended there, as Andrew seemed fine with my responses. He was obviously trying to find out if all things were equal in the family.

As many recipient parents have discovered, getting information about their children's donor is not always easy. There are some forward-thinking clinics who will offer to give all the information they have on the donor when parents conceive a child. Other clinics wait until parents ask. Asking is not always a stress-free thing for recipient parents, especially those who conceived their child in a time when the message coming from medical professionals was 'don't tell anyone.' The fears can range from, 'If I ask will they get angry with me?' to 'Will they give me what I ask for and will they understand why I need the information?'

When our third child, Elizabeth, was less than a year old, Patrice and I wrote to the two clinics we had dealt with requesting information about our children's donors. For me a request in writing was the easiest emotionally but it was still not without fear.

When the letter came from the clinic with details of Andrew's donor, I was petrified as I opened it that they would refuse to give me any information, and in a fleeting moment I imagined trying to tell Andrew that we only knew the colour of the donors eyes, his weight and his height. When I read the letter I was relieved that they were giving us information but I felt depressed that it was so little. All we were told were his physical characteristics, that he had completed tertiary education, was a bank manager, his religion and what his IQ was. My immediate feeling was, 'So that's where Andrew gets his interest in money from,' and, 'Doesn't this person think a lot of himself to put down his IQ.' I felt no closer to this person who had donated his sperm in order to create a life. There was more I wanted to know, his interests, his hobbies, and his outlook on life. And I wondered that if I was having these thoughts how would Andrew feel when he becomes old enough to understand?

We also got information on Callum's and Elizabeth's donors. We knew what year they were born, if they were married or single when they donated, what job they did and what some of their interests were.

We now had some donor information for all three of our children. When we saw the information written down it was a pitifully small amount to describe the men who helped to create our children – we wished that there was more. Why did these men donate? Do they ever wonder about the children they helped to create? We found it sad that what we knew about these very important people could be written down in just a few lines.

Many people may wonder why we applied for this information when our children were still so young and had asked virtually no questions. One reason was that, at that time, clinics in our state were only legally bound to keep information on donors for ten years. We felt that it was our responsibility to make sure that we at least had some information on their donors in our safe keeping. How awful would it be for our children to want information on their donors only to be told that it had been destroyed, and that we knew it could happen and had done nothing to secure even a small amount of information for them?

Just before his ninth birthday Andrew asked if we knew the name of his donor (something he had asked before). Again, we said that we didn't know, and he responded with, 'We'll probably never know.' He asked if we knew anything about the donor and we decided that it was time we showed him the letter we had got from the clinic in response to our request for information on the donor. It took me some time to find the letter. I had filed it safely away in a folder and looked through the folder about three times before I found it. I was quietly panicking, thinking, 'How could I do this to my child, lose such important information?' But I did find it and we all read it together. Andrew wanted to know what the weight range meant and how tall the donor was compared to his dad. We read through the religion of the donor, his education level and that he was a bank manager. After that Andrew said that he thought he was a bit like the donor in build and that he liked money too!

One of the greatest fears that a recipient parent can have when requesting donor information for their child is that they will be told the records have been destroyed. Leonie experienced this when she contacted a clinic about donor information.

> The clinic said that the records for our eldest child no longer existed. I raised this issue with a doctor from another clinic and she had said to me that she found it very difficult to believe as the clinic where she worked kept every donor record since they began their programs. I kept that little bit of information in the back of my mind for about two years until I became confident enough to think about it and deal with it. My clinic was saying that the records don't exist, but I had this doctor telling me that records do exist at her clinic. We (Warren and I) have to clarify this. And we have to tell our children we tried, it's really important to tell our children that we tried to get their information.

It was very important to our family to get the acknowledgment in black and white that they didn't have Geraldine's records. I wanted it in writing that there were no records. I wanted to be able to say to Geraldine, 'This is the letter that says there are no records.' We tried to figure out how Geraldine would feel. She might think, 'Mum says there are no records but how does she know?'

I think we told Geraldine right from the start, that there were no records. She was very angry about that because her sister Genevieve's records were there. She said that it was, 'Very unfair, why should she have it and not me.' I felt sad for my daughter.

We tried on numerous occasions to find more information on Geraldine's donor. We wrote to hospital ethics committees and had a meeting with the CEO and medical director of the hospital, just basically to try to find if Geraldine's records did exist. This process took three or four years, if I remember correctly. We have now established that there are records that identify Geraldine's donor.

Maybe the message here is to persevere and that has also been the case with us when we wanted clinics to contact our three children's donors.

When our children were seven, four, and a year old we wrote letters of thanks to our three donors and gave them a little bit of information on each child. We felt that they might have some curiosity about the children they helped to conceive, and as we had a small amount of information on each of them felt it only fair that they knew something about our children.

The two clinics where we conceived our children had never had a request like ours before and both had to think for quite a while about how they would handle it. Even though donor anonymity has never been written into any laws in most countries, it has been an almost universal practice among infertility clinics. These two clinics we were dealing with seemed to feel that by passing on our letters they could in some way be breaking their promise of anonimity to the donors. One clinic took about a year before they finally decided to contact the donor and ask him if he would receive our letter about Andrew. A little while later they told us that they had been unable to find Andrew's donor. When Andrew asked us about this we told him what had happened, and he didn't seem too bothered by it. I asked him why he wanted to know where the donor was and his reply was, 'Curiosity, he's my physical father.' We had never used the term 'father' when referring to the donor so it certainly showed that

Andrew was beginning to understand more about his relationship to his donor. The other clinic was quicker to contact Callum and Elizabeth's donors but the news was not all good. Callum's donor had moved address and they were unable to locate him. Elizabeth's donor agreed to receive our letter.

About a year later we got a call from the clinic counselor telling us that she had a letter from Elizabeth's donor, would we like to receive it? To say that this was a surprise would be an understatement; we had never asked any questions of him, so for him to write to us of his own accord was wonderful. We got the letter and it was lovely. He told us about his own family background and his own children. He offered to answer any questions that Elizabeth or we might have in future. We felt that Elizabeth was and still is far too young to read this letter but we have put it away safely for the time being. While receiving this letter was joyful, it also carried with it sadness – sadness that our two sons could not have the same thing.

Thoughts of all this was put to the backs of our minds for a while as our family grew, but late last year Andrew saw an advertisement on television for a show on DI where a girl met her donor. Andrew made a note of when it would be on and made sure that we were all sitting down to watch it. After it was finished both Andrew and Callum asked if there was any way they could know the name of their donors. We reminded them that the clinics had not been able to find their two donors but we then asked them if they would like us to write back to the clinics and try again. Callum and Andrew both thought that this would be a good idea so that is what we did. We asked each of the clinics if they could instigate a more thorough search, perhaps involving the electoral rolls, and we were very pleasantly surprised when both clinics agreed to try again.

It has turned out that both our son's donors have now been located. Andrew's donor did not want contact, but the clinic counselor talked to him and with his agreement wrote down a huge amount of information about him – right down to his favourite food. Andrew knows that we have this information but has not asked to read it as yet. Callum's donor also did not want contact and unfortunately the clinic scientist who made contact with him, as far as we know, did not ask for any extra information from him.

What do we do now? Do we accept that Elizabeth and Andrew have quite a bit of information on their donors and Callum has virtually nothing in comparison? Do we just hope that it doesn't hurt our son too much? I know if I were in Callum's shoes I would be very angry at the inequality of it. I would naturally want what my brother and sister had. I think we will let things stay this way for a while and then try again. The donor might change his mind about further contact. With clinics getting more and more requests like ours they may make the counselor responsible for contacting donors and they may be able to request updated information.

There are a growing number of parents like us who also want to make contact with their child's donor. Pam and David talk about what they did.

> We do know a little about Lachlan's donor. We would love to meet him. We wrote a letter to him and sent a photo of the three of us, and we received a positive reply. We don't want him to become a long lost relative but if one day we could bring him along to a support group picnic, that would be just great.
>
> I wish we could meet him to ask a million questions – did he collect rocks as a kid and place them in straight lines according to size and colour? Does he watch any sport and love fishing? I don't do any of these. If Lachlan ever meets him I want to be there. I hope he does one day. (David)

> We asked the clinic if we could write to the donor and what the procedure was. The counselor wrote back and said, 'If you give me a letter, we'll try and contact the donor for you.' She contacted the donor and asked if he would receive a letter from us, and he kindly said yes. He was a bit shocked, because he was told by the clinic that his sperm was not good enough and he was under the impression that it was thrown away. The counselor said that he was a bit overwhelmed to find there's three kids, so we left it a little while. We thought maybe he just needs to get used to the idea – and his family as well because he's got teenage kids. Then we sent off a letter and a photograph of our family and promptly received a positive reply with a photo of the donor. (Pam)

Rose was the first person I ever talked to who had been able to write to her child's donor.

> During treatment, anytime I struck a new member of staff I would enquire further about the donor. Initially we were just given height and

hair colour but there was quite a bit of other non-identifying information on file. Through simple questioning I now had more of a profile on our donor. I then wrote to the clinic social worker and proposed that a questionnaire style letter be sent to the donor to answer. He did reply, and answered our questions in a humorous and honest manner. 'Do you have braces on your teeth? Can you play a musical instrument?' These were the type of questions.

We wrote again asking for a few thoughts from him to be kept and given to our children. He wrote, 'Here I sit at the computer, what do I say that is profound?' He wrote at length, even mentioning his interest in bicycle riding and triathlons. I have written to the counselor to find out how many babies from our donor have made it into the world, and at the last count it was 11. Eleven babies for a maximum of ten families.

To know the donor was prepared to write to us was enormously reassuring. I feel now that I can 'let go', and should our children need some written contact with our donor then it is up to them.

One of the more difficult things that recipient parents have to face about having used donated gametes is the strong possibility of half-siblings. Clinics in a number of countries have guidelines limiting the use of one donor. In the UK, the code of practice that clinics must follow is that a donor must no longer be used once the number of children born from his or her gametes reaches ten. This code has been in place only since the early 1990s, and suggestions have been made that the number of children born from one donor in earlier days was many times higher. In Australia, the limit is ten families (plus the donor's own). So, the total number of donor children alone could easily be twenty or more. The idea of about twenty children out there who are half-brothers and half-sisters to your own child may not be so easy to contemplate.

I found out that the donor has helped to create about nineteen boys and two girls. I feel sad, as though that's a negative, I don't know why. It feels like it belittles my son or something, as if they are a dime a dozen; don't they realize that he's so special? What would worry me is if from the 20 siblings there were lots of girls and that Lachie would meet one. That is an issue. I actually have a lot of detail about the siblings, I have the birth dates, the sexes, and I know how many families. It means that if I ever got that doubtful feeling that another child looks like Lachie I can always check the birth dates. The more knowledge I have the better. I'll keep all this for Lachie and it will probably make him feel better as well. They say

> the chance of half-siblings meeting is unlikely but we all live in a small area. I don't rule it out at all, I think it's quite likely. (Bridget)

Many clinics in countries like Australia will tell parents how many half-siblings there are and whether they are boys or girls, and in what year they were born. Mary has thought a lot about this aspect of donor conception.

> It seems extraordinary that they're focusing so much on the donor information and not on the half-siblings because I'm sure that would be something that the child would be curious about. They might want to know those children, too. They've got just as much right to meet and know those children as they do to meet and know the donor. Funnily enough, for me it's less threatening than them meeting the donor themselves. In other words, I wouldn't find an attachment to a half-sibling threatening, it would seem quite natural and normal. I grew up in a big family. The half-siblings, they're all in the same position as the child really, they weren't in any way involved in the decision that was made on their behalf, they are the result of the decision. They might like to know how each fared and what it was like for them. They are the sort of questions they couldn't really discuss with me because I wouldn't understand that, I couldn't even hope to, really.

Karen contacted the clinic she went to and found out about the number of half-siblings that her son might have.

> Because I've been pregnant again (with my second husband) Brad has had questions like, 'What was it like when you were pregnant with me, how did you feel?' He's curious to know what the donor looks like, he'd like a photo and he would like to write to him. I've got the non-identifying information on the donor so I got that piece of paper out and read it to him.
>
> We found out Brad's donor has six donor children, they're all around the same age, nine, ten or eleven. I thought that's great, Brad knows he's got a few half-brothers or half-sisters. That was his main question, probably because he didn't have any brothers or sisters from me until this new baby. He wanted to know if there was anybody out there who might look like him. If Brad ever wants to get in contact with the donor, I'll do whatever it takes, do whatever he wants me to do. They said for me to keep waiting for him to ask questions but he does want to write to the donor and he does want to write to the children. I said that I would get on

to that again for him, I want to do it in case the donor dies or whatever, we may as well start now, before it's too late.

Like Karen, an increasing number of parents I have spoken to over the years have expressed their willingness to help their children make contact or even meet their donor, if that is their wish.

> I would absolutely go out of my way to satisfy my son's want to find his natural father, I'd help him. In fact, in many ways I have a very special relationship with Jack because of the way he was conceived and because we are now separated. I'm sure the day will come when he will want to find out about his natural father, but I think I've been doing a pretty good job up till now. For all intents and purposes, Jack is my natural son. (Rob)

> If Jake wanted to meet his donor I couldn't stop him, I wouldn't feel 100 percent about it but I would still let him. It's his business and if it's what he wants to do I'd help him. (Paul)

> I think that I would have to give him every help that he needed because if I don't, not only is it his right but he could hold it against me. I have no choice really. Not that I wouldn't want to help because the evidence says that despite the fact that the other person is the biological father Paul will always be his real father, so it's not really that scary. (Barbara)

> I've thought a lot about whether they might want to meet the donor and I think I'm at the stage now where I'd be happy and I'd like them to be curious. If they didn't ever say that they wanted to meet the donor I might just feel they were keeping it inside and they don't want to tell me because they don't want to upset me. I'd help them in any way I could to find the donor. I think it would be a good thing for them to meet him, and for me. I'd like to thank him, as it was a pretty good thing to do. (Julian)

> I'd probably like to meet him, I feel a certain amount of curiosity, I want our children to know that they have our complete support if they want to meet the donor. I would be very surprised if neither of them want to know. I think I might almost be a little bit disappointed if they don't. I won't encourage them in that direction or try to influence them either way but I guess I expect to have that happen one day. There's also the whole issue of if the donor can't be contacted and how we will deal with that. When I last checked with the clinic I think there were four half-siblings. (Janet)

> I'm very comfortable with them trying to find out as much information as they want about their donors. My overriding consideration is what they want; it's not what I want. If they want to find out information or have some sort of communication with the donor in writing or phone conversations, or if they want to meet the donor, whatever makes them happy is what will make me happy. (Warren)

There are of course a very few parents and offspring around the world who have actually met with their donors. Earlier in this chapter I mentioned an Australian television program which looked at a young girl who had been able to meet her donor, and she and her family had established a relationship with the donor and his wife. There are also a number of cases of older offspring in Australia who have been able to meet their donors. Becky, who lives in the US, tried to make contact with the two donors who helped to create her three children.

> It was my impetus, and not theirs. From watching what they were going through, it made me want to contact the donors for more information. All we really had were vital stats. Brandon, for instance, was slow in gaining height. I know many people still gain height in college, I wanted to give him hope that that was in store for him. He also had developed a profound focus on baseball. I contacted a counselor for people thinking of using DI and asked her of any questions that in her experience might come up later. She said, inevitably they want to know why the donor became a donor. I liken this to the adoption question of 'Why did you give me up?' Another impetus to me was an adopted girl at work who had just found her biological parents only to find that her biological dad died in an automobile accident when she was very young. I was concerned that the longer I waited, the more difficult it might be to find the man, or he may have suffered an untimely death and we would never find him.
>
> I first talked with the twins' donor in March of last year. He came here in June. Before he came, we tried to anticipate issues to make everyone as comfortable as possible. What to call [the donor] was an issue for a number of weeks. There aren't enough endearing words in the English language to have something special for each person. We drifted from friend, to special friend, to distant relative, and finally I decided he was their father, but not their dad. He didn't fill the 'Dad' role. However, Lins decided later, on her own, [the donor] was her dad. She casually said it was pretty special to have two dads. In August, we went to meet [the

donor's] family. I was tremendously impressed by their open-mindedness and warmth, particularly of [the donor's] eighty-five year old father. My kids had never had a relationship with someone that age before and it was a plus for all of us. Nearly immediately, he told me he hoped the kids would come to call him Opa [German for 'grandpa']. Unfortunately, we lost him in January of this year.

I have had a rough time with a couple of issues in all of this. First was to determine how I relate to [the donor]. Not many people can say they had someone's children but never were intimate with them. There is an undeniable bond. I finally decided there are many kinds of love and I don't love my children as I do my friends. I decided I loved [the donor] in a special way all his own. After we each went to the other's homes to visit, there was no more mention of future meetings and I got very nervous that the curiosity had been satisfied and I had made a huge mistake in opening my children up to someone who may not want to stay connected. Luckily, [the donor] has better-than-average male communication skills and we were able to talk through that to some degree. When you have had two men to leave you and your children's lives, you don't want them hurt again.

Brandon (my oldest) and I are 'together' on the relationship with the twins' donor. He is our friend. He is the twins' father. We have decided that 'family' can be anyone you want it to be and the more friends, the better. Brandon is more impacted by my two failed marriages than he is by having a new friend. The twins' donor has been very good at including Brandon and doing things with him too (and Brandon notices).

Of course, there are going to be hundreds of thousands of donor offspring for whom contact with their donor will never be possible. For the majority, this will be because they have never been told the truth of their conception. For others, it will be for a variety of reasons: the clinic cannot find the donor, the donor does not want contact, or the donor records have been destroyed. This last reason is a distinct possibility for many donor offspring conceived 15 to 20 years ago – especially those conceived in a time when fresh semen was used. Unfortunately, it may also apply to some much younger offspring whose parents attended clinics that have not yet understood the importance of retaining donor records.

The parents and offspring who have very little chance of getting donor information or making contact with their donor do not always sit back and accept things the way they are. There are a number of people in this situation who are working to make things better for others, such as Anne in Canada.

> I feel we have a close relationship today because I was truthful and didn't break the bonds of trust and honesty between parent and child. I wrote the doctor, who gave me sparse information back and expressed his lack of memory of who our donor was. I don't believe he kept any accurate records and that is why I work so hard to change the system for future generations and to show Mae that I did the best I could to make things better for the offspring.

11

Discussion with Donor Offspring

I saw a newspaper article, 'Donor Dad Meets his Son.' I thought, 'My God, there's other people like me.' I had thought I was the only one. (Priscilla)

Children do not ask to be born nor do they have any choice in the method of their conception. I, like many other parents who have conceived our children using donated gametes, wonder what my children will think about their conception as they grow. Will they hate me for using an anonymous donor? Will they spend their lives wondering who this man is and trying to find him? Will the non-identifying information that they have about their donors and the knowledge that they were desperately wanted satisfy them as they grow? In other words, will love be enough?

My own children are still too young for me to have in-depth conversations about what donor conception means to them as individuals, so all I have to go on is my conversations with adults that I am in contact with who were born by donor insemination. Through talking to them many thoughts have passed through my mind about how donor conception is practiced including, should only known or identifiable donors be allowed to donate? To this my answer is a resounding 'yes'. Should parents and donors have to meet before the conception of a child? A scary thought for many but perhaps it is a way of reinforcing the reality of what is about to be undertaken. And last, the biggest question of all, should donor conception be allowed to continue at all?

The people who have been wonderful enough to talk to me and write of their experiences for use in this chapter and the next are a very wide-ranging group of people. They come from four different countries: Australia, the US, the UK and Canada. They range in age from those in their teenage years to those in their fifties, and all were born from sperm provided by an anonymous man. Some were told about the method of their conception at quite a young age while others were told or found out when they were teenagers, adults or into their middle years. Some have a little bit of non-identifying information about their donor but most know nothing at all.

Lauran, Shelley and Mae were told by their parents when they were quite young.

> Mum was still breastfeeding Ian, my younger brother, and I asked where babies come from and she told me. She showed me a book about DI conception, that was when I was about four or four-and-a-half. I'm not sure if I asked any questions – it was sort of, 'Yeah, OK.' A couple of years later (it's never been a subject we haven't talked about in the house) Paul Keating (then Prime Minister of Australia) just happened to be on the news and I said, 'Could he be my father?' (Lauran)

> My mom told me when I was seven years old that I was born by AI. We had just watched a program on TV about DI and she asked me what I thought about it. Then we talked some more about it and she told me. My immediate reactions were, 'Hey, now I know why my mom always told me I was worth thousands to her.' (I should note that when I asked her about this she laughed and said that was only one of the reasons, the other was that the saying is metaphorical.) From a very young age I was convinced that I was adopted, and so when my mom told me that I was born by DI it finally made sense. (Shelley)

> When I was five I started to ask my mom how babies were made. She told me about the sperm and the egg, and continued further to tell me my own story of how I was made. She said my dad didn't have enough sperm, so 'Daddy and I went to see a kind doctor, who gave us the sperm of a man who had extra and wanted to help people who couldn't have babies.' (Mae)

Brigitte and Barry were both told in their teenage years.

> I remember not knowing how to feel, I wanted to know what it was all about, as I didn't know what they were going on about. Then my sister and I had a game of chess with our dad, and when I went to bed I remember crying. (Brigitte)

I was eighteen. My dad had died that summer. Our mother told us nervously on Christmas Eve. It was fine. I appreciated her doing so. (Barry)

Priscilla found out in her very late teens, but the situation was not a good one.

I got married at the age of eighteen and by the time I was nineteen I already had my first child, Hayley, who is now eight. At the time my mum and dad were separated. There was a family fight and Mum threatened to tell us but Dad beat her to it. He knocked on my front door and said, 'I've got something to tell you. I'm not your real dad, your mum was artificially inseminated.' My first reaction was, 'I know,' but deep inside I really didn't. I had no idea. I always thought I might have been adopted or something like that but never ever thought that this was how I came about. After being told, the jigsaw sort of fitted together. When there was anything on TV about IVF, Mum and Dad would always speak in Dutch together. There were little hints there but I didn't put the pieces together until I was told. At the time I said that it didn't matter, that it didn't make any difference. I really tried to push it to the back of my mind, I really wanted to just forget about it, it was just too hard for me to deal with.

Barry also did not suspect the truth.

We were what you might call distant in emotional style. We were English, though, and that is common. My father was not close to me. I never suspected anything like DI, though.

For many people like Priscilla and Barry the news of their biological identity can come as a huge shock. They have believed for so many years that they are blood relatives of both their parents and suddenly, in the blink of an eye, this has changed.

The immediate thoughts that have gone through people's minds on being told this momentous news are many and varied. While Sherrie-Lee had not suspected the truth of her conception she had noticed differences between herself and her dad.

I thought that it was kinda sad, 'cause I originally thought I was just born and made like everyone else was. As most kids do when they are growing up I asked my mum and dad if I was adopted, because I had noticed that I looked nothing like my dad. One day I remember saying to him, 'How come my thumbs aren't like yours?' I think back now to that question and wonder what Dad would have been thinking, because for me to have asked that I expect would have hurt Dad's feelings, even though I didn't know I wasn't his biological child.

My parents told me and my younger sister when I was just starting year ten (almost fifteen). One of the first things I remember thinking to myself was, 'Who is my real biological father?' I'm still interested and one day hope to get the chance to meet him and find out everything about him. When Mum and Dad told us it didn't sink in for a while because it was too hard to believe. Everything was new and confused. That night I cried myself to sleep, asking myself, 'Why me?' The next day was the hardest because I treated Dad different and that lasted for two weeks. Me and my sister cope with things differently so she did not treat Dad any differently.

Feelings will inevitably evolve over time. Issues emerge that were not obvious to start with.

I felt sad that my dad wasn't really half me. I also felt frustrated that I didn't know who my biological dad was. I have asked my mum and dad questions like, 'Can I find out who my biological dad is? Would I have other half-brothers and half-sisters? Is my sister my real sister? Why couldn't my dad make babies?'

I would like to know about my donor and what he looks like. I would also like to know if I have other half-brothers and half-sisters and if so, where they are, what they look like, what are they like, do they know about how they were conceived?

I know that my parents had a lot of trouble getting me. They did everything they could and in the end they got me because they wanted me so much. I feel extra special and very loved by them.

I feel that the education department should teach about this stuff in health so that kids at school don't make jokes about it because they don't understand it. If they understood it they would realize that the jokes they make about it are silly and don't really make sense. It hurts me when they joke about it. (Brigitte)

Overall, I don't believe my knowing of my conception has affected my relationships with family and friends with the exception of my father. Because I have always known the truth of my conception my relationship with my mother has always been as it is. The DI is a part of who I am. My knowing my conception is a complete non-issue with other family members and friends, it's who I am, like the colour of my hair, and I don't think it has made a difference on the types of relationships we have developed.

My father, on the other hand, is a different story. I believe he never fully dealt with his infertility before going through with the DI procedure. As I was growing up I was a constant reminder of this fact. My knowing the truth has affected our relationship, because once I knew the truth, he couldn't deny the procedure or his infertility, which is something he would rather forget. (Mae)

Anything I try to discuss with Dad he just does not want to talk about, he gets really angry and sort of hurt, he's really, really threatened. I respect him and love him more than before because it takes someone special to bring up a child who's not genetically theirs. When I did talk to my mother she said, 'We weren't allowed to tell you.' But since then she's said, 'Oh, that person already knows,' and I think how come it was good enough for them to know but not for me to know? What was wrong with me knowing? She can't answer me.

Some days when I look in the mirror I think this is just too hard, it must have been a mistake, Mum got artificially inseminated but perhaps it was really Dad's sperm. It's easier to think that way than to think that someone donated sperm to enable my conception. I asked Mum and because Dad had no sperm at all, it was donor sperm. But there is still that little bit of hope; it would just be so much easier.

When I first got pregnant with Madison (my fourth child) I was really emotional and it all started coming out. I was looking at my own children and thinking, 'Oh my God, they've got parts of me but where did I get them from?' I now have five children aged between ten years and ten months and feel it is unfair that I don't have the human right to know my biological father. (Priscilla)

Other than going to meetings and outings with the group (DCSG), here in Western Australia nothing else in my life has changed. I still feel the same, act the same, and think the same. Having friends and family to support me has helped me through the past four years that I have known that I am a donor child. I see being a donor child as something special and different and I'm very lucky to be here. And I would like to thank my mum and dad for going to all the trouble of having me, and I love them both very much for that. (Sherrie-Lee)

A question that is being asked more and more frequently is how the children of single women and same-sex couples feel about their donors. Is it any different from those children raised in a family with both a mother and a father? Shelley's mother was single when she used DI.

> I have never thought negatively about the way I was born, I have always felt special. And I love other people's reactions when I tell them how I was born. They always react with the same: 'Cool, that is so neat, I've never met anyone born by AI before.' My thoughts have always been that I am truly special and that I was born because my mom really wanted a child. I am proud to be who I am. I don't think that it made any difference that I did not have a dad around while I was growing up. My mom has always been my mom and my dad. She cooks, she cleans, she is the sole breadwinner, but she also builds things, repairs vehicles and electronics. She bakes homemade bread, but she mows the lawn while waiting for it to rise. I could never replace the 'dad' in my mom, only add a new dad to my life. I don't think the fact that I did not have a dad around made me think differently about the donor. I know of a pair of sisters who both think differently than me and they were both born by AI. One doesn't care and the other wants to know, but not nearly as badly as I do. I think that it just all depends on the person. (Shelley)

Once told about their origins donor offspring may feel the need to tell others.

> The next day (after being told) I rode to my best friend's house and told her. It was hard to get it out because it was all new to me too. She asked questions but I couldn't answer them 'cause I didn't know the answers. It was good to tell someone, as I needed to talk about it. I chose my best friend because I didn't feel comfortable talking with Mum and Dad. I told my other best friend in year 11 and by then I knew the answers to her questions because I had been going to the DCSG meetings and outings, which made things easier as I was with other donor children and being there made it easier to ask Mum and Dad questions. Lately I have told more friends and it makes it easier for me that my closest friends know all about my past. Some answers I still don't have but if I want to know it's easy to find out if you have parents that don't mind answering questions and discussing the topic of donor conception. (Sherrie-Lee)

I have been selective when deciding who to tell of my conception. I have told a few friends over the years but only those who I feel truly respect me and are mature in their outlook on life. I don't believe I'm viewed differently when they know of the situation. Quite often I think most of the issues go over their heads. (Mae)

Friends at school, they were like, 'Oh, wow!' That was when I was younger, now all my friends know and they can't understand why more people don't know about it. Talking with friends, who only know what I've told them, they don't understand how it's any different from adoption, and quite frankly I can't either. (Lauran)

Lauran and her friends have made a connection between donor conception and adoption, as have many others. They've also noticed the fact that, while adoption records are able to be accessed legally by adoptees, that right does not extend to donor offspring trying to get even non-identifying information about their donors.

We've discussed in previous chapters about parents requesting information on donors from clinics but there are also donor offspring who have searched for information themselves. Lauran wrote to the clinic that her parents had attended, and was originally told that there was no information. She persisted and wrote a second letter.

In the second letter they only gave me one-and-a-half lines [of donor information] it was really disheartening.

I don't know whether betrayed is the right word; I was lied to when they said there was no information. The letter gave me his height, (so I've got no hope of ever being tall because he's only 5 foot 6), his hair colour, and his eye colour. He was a uni. student when he donated and that gave me a rough idea of his age, so you can sketch up some sort of image. There's eight offspring to him, me included.

I've written letters since asking for mainly medical history, any information at all. I really want his medical history, any hobbies, any interests, right down to his shoe size, basically.

Priscilla has spent a lot of time and emotional energy trying to find some information about her donor.

When I first started searching for information I went through numerous phone books to try and find out about the clinic my mum went to. I got in touch with the doctor's wife and she told me that the records had been destroyed when the doctor stopped practicing in 1979. She said that they were destroyed to protect the donors' identity. I found the clinic receptionist who could remember Mum taking me back to see the doctor when I was two. She said she could remember my brown eyes and my little round face. We had a quick chat and she was amazed that I ever found out. She rang me back about two weeks later and said, 'Look Priscilla, you've got two beautiful parents who love you and want you and needed you, this isn't what it was meant to be. You weren't meant to search for the donor. It was an anonymous donation.' I thought, 'Can't anyone understand what I'm going through?' Then I doubted myself and thought, 'What am I doing this for?', but I got on top of it.

It's vital information, for my own identity. I really do need to know because it just eats at me. It doesn't matter where I look or what I do it's always there niggling me. I always thought there might be a cure for the way I feel and hopefully it would heal over. I have since learned that I will always have to deal with these unknown ghosts about myself. I will continue my search for the truth until I find it. It is a burden which is heavy; I can only hope this does not affect other people the way it has affected my life, me as a person. Now people know the effects secrecy holds and cannot say they didn't know this would happen.

I saw my dad recently, and on the way home I had tears running down my face because I'd asked him to come on a television show with me to talk about donor conception and he refused and was really angry. I'm not doing this to hurt him, I love him with every cell of my body, but I just need to know. It's so frustrating because it's not only my needs but it's my dad's and my mum's, I've got to think of all of those people. It's really torturing, I can't think of another word to describe it.

After talking to a number of adult offspring I found that many feel they have to perform this very delicate balancing act that Priscilla has described. They can be curious about their donor or have a need to find out information about him but they also feel, often quite deeply, that by having these thoughts and trying to satisfy their curiosity they may in some way be hurting the parents who have raised them. However, there are also adult offspring who have their parents' support in seeking information about their biological origins.

I have always been very close to my mom. Perhaps because of the way I was born, but more likely because it has always been her and me, no one else. I am an only child and when I was younger she never had girl-friends, or at least not to my knowledge! My mother and I have always been very close, and I imagine we always will be, regardless of whether I find my father or not. She supports my search and stands behind me all the way. She knows that it is nothing against her, as I love her to death, but it is something that I need to do for me.

The only information that I have on my donor is his basic statistics, height, weight, eye and hair colour, blood type, and that he was a med. student at Vancouver General Hospital in Canada at the time of donation. I have no knowledge of any half-siblings, I don't think that the clinic would tell me.

I have been searching in vain for my father for about five years now, and will continue the search until I find him or I die. It means everything to me to find my father. Family is so very important to me, and although he isn't really my 'dad,' I would still love to know about him. (Shelley)

At the beginning of this chapter I posed the question, 'Should donor con-ception be allowed to continue?' For those involved in the area it is a very difficult question often loaded with complex emotions. Donor conception is a money-making concern, and if it was banned medical professionals working in reproductive technology would lose a percentage of their incomes. For recipient parents to talk about stopping the practice of donor conception can be seen as selfish by some, along the lines of, 'It's alright for you, you have your children.' Recipient parents may also worry that, by considering stopping the practice of donor conception, children may feel that their parents wish they had never been born, and this is certainly very far from the truth.

For offspring to voice an opinion on banning donor conception can be emotionally charged as well. They risk the ire of infertile people who may accuse them of not understanding the pain of infertility. They may also worry how their views will affect their own parents who used this method of reproductive technology to conceive them.

I believe DI should still be allowed to be practiced in Canada. However, with the current 'system' the doctor's are under no obligation to be accountable to anyone or keep accurate up-to-date records. It is these two issues that I believe must be changed. I also believe the offspring should have the right to see their records when they come of age. (Mae)

It should be allowed to continue, but donors should have to agree to be identifiable. There should be a document in addition to a birth certificate, perhaps, that lists the donor(s). Identifiability would probably best come upon the maturity of the child. (Barry)

If I'm faced with infertility, there's no way I could ever go through with DI. (Lauran)

12

Thoughts and Experiences of Donor Offspring

Louise (UK)

I was told about my conception three years ago at the age of 32, when I was on holiday with my mum – Dad had stayed home. The disclosure was entirely unpremeditated on my mum's part. We were talking about some of the emotional stuff I'd been going through, and she just knew that she had to tell me the truth. It was obviously traumatic for both of us, but it was strangely peaceful too – the truth is always liberating, and though, yes, it was a shock to me, it resonated as truth at such a deep level that it was almost as if I'd always known. I felt immediately freed into being who I am – though it has taken the last three years even to begin to work out in practice what that means. It was also as if the bottom dropped out of my world, as all the familiar parameters disappeared. The feelings were very complex. I felt intense sadness for my dad, that he hadn't had his own natural kids, compassion for my mum, who'd lived with a painful secret for so many years, euphoria and despair all mixed together for myself. I felt sad that I wasn't related to my dad in light of his good qualities – and relief in light of some of his not-so-good ones, and his failure often to understand me intuitively.

Hot on the heels of the sadness and compassion came anger, which took a year or so to work out – I was furious at him for tying me up in knots (not deliberately), as I'd striven so hard to please him and to be like him, and never known the reason why it never seemed to work.

As for whether I'd sensed anything different about our family, the answer is 'yes and no.' Certainly not consciously. I never suspected I was adopted – I am very like my mother, physically, emotionally, and intellectually, and also like her side of the family – whom I only met when I was

27 as they're all overseas. I had simply assumed that her genes had been extremely dominant! Dad and I used to joke about the tiny ways in which we are similar – particularly the fact that we have the same weirdly-shaped little fingers! I had no idea at the time what a bitter-sweet joke it was. But there were intense pressures and stresses in our family life, and now I know the extent to which the secret of my conception was a part of that – though not the only cause, by any means. I think subconsciously I must have known more. I used to go to church with my parents and think, 'How strange that I'm his daughter and all these other people aren't.' At the time, I put that down to the fact that he has a very fatherly heart towards people in general, and I considered myself privileged to be his daughter, but with hindsight it was a very strange thing to think – I never thought, 'How strange that she's my mother' – she just was! I also remember one day saying to my dad, 'If we weren't related, I don't think we'd naturally be friends' – I think I must have been somewhere between 12 and 15. That must have nearly killed him. I probably still feel a measure of that insecurity in the relationship. I know he loves me – he's shown it consistently in word and deed all my life, and all he's said since he's known I know is that he wouldn't change anything, and the past thirty-five years have been a delight and treasure to him. We have a good friendship, and I think I'm beginning to find a genuine deep love towards him again in my heart. But I am still somewhat insecure – I just don't know if he would actually like me as a person if there were no adoptive connection between us. Maybe I just need to ask him.

My life has been transformed since knowing the truth. My current flatmate has known me for many years – before and after – and she cannot get over the difference! Knowing the truth of who I am (even though, of course, I only know half of my genetic origins) has unleashed a level of confidence I never dreamed possible. Admittedly, it's not only the truth about my conception that's changed things. Mum's revelation coincided with my leaving a long-term and very unsatisfying job with a generous redundancy pay-out, which has funded me to begin a new life, doing some of the things I have always longed to do. Part of that has been pursuing my Christian faith in a new way, and receiving some excellent prayer-counseling (about DI and other issues) which has touched me at a deep level, bringing a new level of spiritual, emotional and psychological wholeness into my life. The knowledge of who I am, however, is central to all this. I'm finally at liberty to set about discovering the real me.

Telling other people the truth about myself is definitely part of the normalizing process. The first year or so was terrible, as Mum was pretty paranoid about anybody knowing. Going overseas for several months has helped, as I've been much freer to make new friends – and share with some old ones – on the basis of my true identity, without it impinging at all on my family at home. In the UK (where I'm from) it's still the case that only a handful of my friends know the truth. I'd like more to know, but I'm sure that will come in time as Mum relaxes more and more on the issue. In some instances it's not just because of my mum's scruples that I've been reticent – a few of my friends would, I fear, react rather oddly! It's wonderful sharing with people who understand where I'm coming from – who grasp the magnitude, but also don't elevate it to the level of some kind of terminal illness. There's nothing worse than trying to talk about something profoundly personal with people who just don't get it! So I've tended to pick and choose quite carefully who I say what to – though I'm getting more casual and laidback about it all the time! The friends I have told have been understanding and supportive – they've absorbed the information, and when I've needed to discuss it they've been willing to, but they have been able to sustain a normal friendship too – I don't want to be known as the 'DI girl.' I'm me, and just happen to be a DI-conceived adult.

I have practically no information on my donor. Mum was told that he was a married, family man, and she had the impression from the clinic that he was a nice bloke! To date I have not made an attempt to find him. When I first knew, I was so distraught at the secrecy, lack of any recourse to information and absence of any support systems, that I didn't consider myself strong enough to start looking. For the first eighteen months to two years, I was desperate to know who he was, but I knew that the desperation would actually leave me very vulnerable were I to start the search on my own. I've actually been biding my time, gambling that things will open up, that gradually the powers-that-be will understand our case and a right of access to records, together with support agencies (official or informal) will be introduced. I have recently found a potential source of information on the clinic at which I was conceived, and I shall gently pursue that, as I'm feeling a lot stronger and less vulnerable now.

As for whether donor conception should continue in its present form, the answer, of course, has to be a resounding no. It's deeply inhumane to put kids together from genetic DIY kits. I'm sorry if that sounds offensive. I fully understand that that is not the motive of DI parents, nor, in many cases, of donors. But it's how it feels. Like bits of you have been grabbed from somewhere, and you have no idea where. I don't particularly care about the niceties of donor anonymity. We are human beings. Human beings are body, soul and spirit, and we come from parents – a mother and a father. In cases where that natural family is pulled apart, for whatever reason, and children are orphaned, abandoned, or rejected, of course adoption is the right, kind, humane course to take. I would never say that only biological bonds are valid – kids growing up in biological nuclear families are often abused or neglected, and receive any true parenting from relationships outside the nuclear, natural family. But DI goes to the opposite extreme and flies in the face of natural genetic bonding, discounting it altogether, turning an in extremis situation like adoption and turning it into a routine practice (I'm aware that I'm probably not making an awful lot of sense!). It steals half their genetic identity from kids. It has to open up: donor anonymity serves only donors. Parents might think it serves them too, but only because of the human propensity to think that if we ignore something it will go away. It's there, whether we acknowledge it or not. At the end of the day, a DI child came from a donor (I use child loosely to refer to any person conceived through DI). Releasing access of information on that donor also releases the child to love, from their heart and their own free will, their adoptive parent. Love is free. Relationships based on truth can be free relationships, and therefore the only ones in which true love can exist.

Bill (US)

Growing up as a person conceived through donor insemination is a difficult experience to describe to anyone who has never had any doubts about their parentage. For infertile people it is even more difficult to understand because of your wishes for your child to grow up secure and comfortable about his self-image. The pain of losing that connection with the child you should have had makes it uncomfortable to think about your child feeling a sense of disconnection from you as his parents. The temptation to keep the truth from your child is extremely compelling because of that fear. Perhaps, if you are an adoptee or a child who never met his father, then you can have some sense of what this is like.

Who am I? Everyone asks that basic question. People form their identities from their childhood experience within families and school, from social interactions, and from other environmental influences. We identify ourselves through our inherent interests, talents, and personalities. A major key to our identity is our genetic blueprint which, for most people, can be read in the faces of parents and extended families and can be seen in the photographs and stories about their ancestors. For adoptees, that essential element in their identity is missing. Total strangers have presumed a godlike power over that vital information, which they consider as irrelevant. Agencies and courts claim the power to protect adoptees by denying access to their birth parents. Adoptees remain eternal children, never gaining the adult autonomy which full identity brings. They live in families that have a visible genetic heritage but it is not their own.

For people conceived through Assisted Reproductive Technologies (ARTs), or DI, the story is identical. We are, in essence, adoptees through donor insemination, donor eggs, surrogacy, or donor embryos. We share the same struggle for full identity, although our circumstances differ in ways that are not as significant as many would have you believe. The people who deny the analogy between DI and adoption know nothing about the lives we live.

Who are the people conceived through ARTs? What is it like to be a DI adoptee? What do we want? Many people have presumed to speak for us, without our permission, without any knowledge of who we are. They have defined us to suit their own bias. Doctors are like fertility gods who view us purely as abstract commodities to assist infertile couples, lesbians, and single women who are unable to have children. They rarely look beyond the microscopic view of gametes, zygotes, blastocysts, embryos, or the ultrasonic images of fetuses, to see the human face of the people they create. Their primary focus has been the pain suffered by their infertility patients. They have not considered the needs of the children who are the central reason for their profession.

Sperm donors are the mysterious participants in this method of family building. Are they more like birth parents who relinquish their children or are they more akin to the deadbeat dads who only care about their immediate pleasure? We know that some of them see their children as a means to perpetuate their genes, to satisfy their biological imperative. We also know that many have a lingering curiosity about our fates. They cannot forget about us after leaving their essence in a beaker at the clinic. However, like other birth parents, they are denied further contact with their future children. Despite that, several of them have actively sought contact with us.

Infertility patients often see us as the fantasy babies they have sought for so long. However, they have a difficult time thinking of the baby as an adolescent, teenager, adult, or the future parents of their grandchildren. It is hard to think of the future when they look at the empty crib in their nursery. DI parents have raised us but, because of the shame they feel about their infertility, they are reluctant to discuss our origins with us, fearful we would reject them for their decision. So, they generally do not disclose. They do not understand that we are undergoing genetic bewilderment. They often suffer from that themselves, raising children whose personalities, traits and feelings are foreign to them, even to the mother who gave them half their genes. They often feel it is unnecessary to disclose the truth of the child's origins, believing that the child/adult will never suspect his or her paternity. When parents decide to be secret, they often delude themselves into believing they can mold us as if we were a blank slate without genetic determinants. Secrecy and deception have built walls between parent and child, creating barriers to full understanding and poisoning the quality of our relationships.

Sociologists have had little success in learning who we are, primarily because DI is so secretive that access to DI families for study is often impossible. Therefore, their view is skewed because their only recourse is generally with DI parents of younger children. They speak with our parents but never with us.

The public has the least information about DI adoptees, as presented through the clouded lens of the media. They see this as a temporary hot issue that only focuses on the pain of the infertile.

How do I see myself? I was born through DI at the end of World War II when the practice of DI was at its utmost level of secrecy. I have an older adopted brother and two younger DI brothers. None of the four separate fathers of these children knew who we were. The man we all called 'Dad' was remote to us emotionally. When I was five years old I became aware of my older brother's adopted status. Naturally, I asked my mother if she adopted me too. She said, 'No, you're my child.' Even at that age, such a response seemed strange to me. The experience of growing up in the shadows of secrecy was at times terrifying. I knew it had something to do with my silently brooding father. I blamed myself for my inability to fit within the pattern he set for me. I tried to be like him and forced myself to watch endless hours of sports and tried out for several athletic teams in school since I felt I could only get his affection that way. He certainly did not seem to appreciate my drawings, the models I built, the classical music I loved to listen to, or the books I read. My failure on the courts and in the fields only amplified my sense of alienation from him. As I became a teenager, I became increasingly aware of the physical dissimilarities between us. In fact, I could not see myself in his face or body at all. I could not see anything in common between my three brothers and me as well. It was as if five total strangers were randomly chosen out of a crowd and told they were a family. Even my brothers' friends looked at me strangely whenever I first met them. My only solace was my mother, who loved to speak with me about our mutual interests in books. However, even she did not understand or nurture my interests in music, dance and art. Much of my personality was at odds with her.

By the time I was in high school, I began to wonder which of our family friends was my true father. I began to feel embarrassed about my mother, feeling she must have been unfaithful to my dad. That thought explained why he seemed to resent me. By the time I graduated, I was so confused about my identity that I had to leave home to restore my failing sanity.

After three years abroad in the Navy, I finally returned home to attend architecture school. The old feelings of confusion returned so I began to spend most of my time away from my family, absorbed in my design studio and courting my future wife. During the next 15 years, I spent less and less time with my parents until my dad's retirement and subsequent declining health. During the final five years of his life, however, we became close at last as he underwent seven progressive amputations of his toes, feet, and legs. He joked that the more I visited him, the less I saw of him. I was acutely aware that our relationship improved once I became a father myself. We spent many intimate hours alone together in the hospital without my mother, and I finally began to feel like his true son.

Only one year after my father's death, my younger brother died as well, from an acute respiratory infection. A week or so later I spent a long afternoon with my mother mourning our recent losses. I began to speak of my fears of inheriting the same infection that claimed my father. By that time in my life, I had totally repressed the certainty he was not my father. My mother gave me a strange look and I was taken aback by the fear I saw in her face. I don't know why I said it, but I finally mentioned that I used to suspect my dad wasn't my genetic father but that I didn't feel that way anymore. She suddenly gave a huge sigh and told me I was conceived through artificial insemination. I did not believe her at first, since I thought DI could not have been more than twenty years old. I was unaware that it began as early as 1884 in the US. I must have been in some kind of shock of denial. As she explained the story to me, every-thing about my earlier confusion started to become clear. I felt a strange mixture of emotions that I cannot adequately describe. I suppose that I was angry at being deceived for so long, but the main effect I felt was a sense of exhilarating liberation. I immediately asked a flurry of questions about the whole process and my mother gave me as much detail as possible, including the name of the OB/GYN [obstetrician/gynaecologist). She told me that my donor graduated from the University of Utah Medical School in 1945, was married and had a daughter. As I pressed for more information in later conversations, my mother began to resent my curiosity. She felt it should have been enough just to know the truth and could not understand my curiosity about the donor who was, after all, my father. Within a few months, she suffered a series of debilitating strokes that left her mostly incoherent, so I was unable to get much more information from her.

After her death six years later, I set out on my quest to identify and meet my donor. The first experience was particularly humiliating since I naively assumed I could just call the clinic and they would give me his name and address. You can probably imagine the response. The receptionist accused my late mother of violating her sacred promise never to tell me about my origins and castigated me for my curiosity that she viewed as a threat to the donor. I did have some information that he had graduated in the class of 1945 at the University of Utah Medical School. I had a list of the 35 graduates and their current addresses from a directory of physicians that could possibly lead to a connection. I met so many dead-ends and spent so many tedious hours searching for photographs that I eventually had to give up because it felt so impossible. I have been unable to muster the energy for a concerted effort.

Instead, I have become an activist for open records and an advocate for disclosure. I have spent much of my time on the Internet on infertility bulletin boards trying to persuade DI parents of the need to disclose. Over the course of the last seventeen years, I have been active in the media as well. I have made contact with over seventy other DI adoptees in Canada, the UK, the US, Australia and now New Zealand. After years of feeling so isolated within my own family, it was immensely reassuring to meet people whose histories were nearly identical to my own. There were so many consistent patterns that I felt that the general public and future recipients of DI needed to understand how our experiences shaped us. Initially, I have received most of my empathy from the adoption support group that I had joined over ten years ago and I have been a member of the American Adoption Congress ever since. They have been the chief source of emotional strength and my validation that my sense of being an adoptee is legitimate. They have given me a sense of kinship. They have not treated me like a freak of medical science but have accepted me as a fellow adoptee.

Since I knew there was so little information about us, I conducted a survey to find out more. This survey, in my humble opinion, is a revealing source of information describing the psychosocial impact of DI on those of us who have lived that experience. My respondents ranged in age from eight years old to fifty-seven. For the most part, they have suffered a great deal from the damage that secrecy created for them during their childhood and the negative effects it had on their parents. Many of those who were not told until adulthood had a strong sense of the secret throughout their childhood. Many suspected their mothers had an affair. All believe that a DI adoptee should be told as early as possible. Those who have been told at an early age have had a substantially happier childhood than the rest of us. However, they are also angry that clinics and governments prevent them from what they perceive as their civil right to know their origins. More than 90 percent feel they have the right to know the donor's identity as well as the right to meet him.

The DI adoptees I know are passionate about their rights, which have been denied them. They are angry at the system that has made them second-class citizens. Within the last year alone, several have initiated their own researches in DI and now refuse to remain invisible. It is my hope that current and future DI parents will understand our need to know the truth at an early age. We also hope that they can find the empathy to support us in our struggle for equal rights of access to our full identity. We are indeed grateful for our lives but feel that our parents need to understand the importance of our needs without feeling threatened by our curiosity about our donors. We are not tracing our roots in order to find replacement fathers. No one would ever replace our parents who raised and nurtured us. Our autonomy as adults, however, depends on the crucial knowledge of our roots.

Christine (UK)

I was already a mother and a grandmother before discovering that I had been conceived by DI, and although the revelation had its greatest impact on me it is clear that there are important ongoing ramifications for all of the current and future members of my family. My husband was surprised by the calm and reasoned way in which I embraced the news about my unnatural conception and would happily admit that initially he probably had more difficulty in accepting the basic fact than I did. Once he had got over his initial disbelief that artificial reproduction was even available when I was born, he was more than ready to explore the implications and was completely attuned to my interest in knowing the actual identity of the person whose genes and character traits I had inherited. He also shared my sense of anger at the secrecy which had surrounded not just my own conception and identity but the whole business of donor insemination for more than sixty years. I have been exceptionally lucky to have had his continued full support and encouragement in everything I have undertaken in respect of donor issues.

Fortunately, I was spared the trauma of being suddenly catapulted into an identity crisis because I had long reasoned that my parentage was not as straightforward as my birth certificate suggested. For twenty years my husband had indulged my idiosyncratic passion for traipsing around overgrown graveyards searching for the long lost members of our joint family tree, and having confirmed that on my paternal side I had been barking entirely up the wrong one, he was more than happy to speculate on the background of my paternal father. Far from being concerned that he didn't know where his wife had come from he was satisfied that my unknown roots were probably from a much less humble source than those that had been officially attributed to me. He reasoned that my real father was definitely somebody rather than a nobody. Such notions were of little comfort to me when finding my biological father was not exactly an option, and I knew that I was unlikely ever to know who that all-important person was (or still is) and why he had chosen to partake in a program of baby making that would see me, his own, undeniable flesh and blood, abandoned into the care of strangers he would never meet.

Our two daughters were already adults at the time of the revelation and, while they may view the mystery of the identity of my unknown donor as intriguing, it has not particularly altered their perception of me. I am still the mother who wiped their noses and smacked their bottoms when they were naughty. Nor have they been unduly concerned by the enforced lack of contact they have had with their donor grandfather as my supposed father had died when I was small; so they had already accepted that their biological link to our paternal line was missing, and it was my step-father who had filled the role of grandad in their lives. They talk about my donor father with an irreverence and complete lack of respect, as to them he is just some old bloke whose only known attribute is an ability to masturbate to order and to catch the ejaculate in a jar. He is perceived as a figure of fun and ridicule rather than as a real person, but his impact on my life and theirs is a more serious concern to them. Both daughters are adamant that I deserve to know who he is, and the current law which prevents all donor offspring and their heirs from having knowledge about their biological ancestry is an unjustifiable breach of basic human rights.

Being aware that many medical conditions are now known to pass genetically from one generation to the next, it was a major concern that a complete lack of knowledge about my sperm donor's family health has put me and my descendants at a distinct disadvantage in terms of early detection of certain types of disease. Perhaps the blame for the otherwise unexplained severe allergy to milk and related products suffered by my two grandsons should be laid at the door of my unknown donor, for who is to say how many generations an aberration may skip before reappearing? I no longer have to be vigilant about the onset of the diabetes which killed my legal father and other members of his family, and I am heartily glad that I hadn't volunteered to take part in ground-breaking medical research in our locality involving people with a family history of diabetes. My involvement could have given false results and impaired the success of the whole research program. I am now aware of the personal danger that my false identity had put me and my unborn children in when, during pregnancy, I had been asked those all important standard questions relating to family illness and had responded with answers that fitted the person I was supposed to be rather than the person I really was.

While my daughters have no great concerns about their own identities they are now more aware of the possible inconsistencies in the identity of the friends and strangers they interact with. My younger daughter is single and currently vets all prospective boyfriends for any possible former DI connection in their family. She is acutely aware that distant cousins could be lurking under any number of disguises. The greatest identity crisis has surprisingly been suffered by my husband. After much consideration of the facts, the various anomalies in his circumstances and some of the strange parallels we have in our lives and experiences, he has felt it necessary to examine the outrageous possibility that he may also have been conceived by DI. If he, too, came out of a little glass jar, would his parents have gone to London for treatment or would they have visited the same clinic as my mother, especially as they lived closer to it than she did? Could we be descended from the same donor? What nonsense, people might think. Lightening doesn't strike twice in the same place! Statistically, the likelihood would be improbable, but then again, how many ordinary working-class mothers in the early 1950s would have owned their own thermometer? With both of his parents now dead and with the clinic records apparently destroyed, there is no way of confirming or invalidating his suspicions.

For the last three years our daughters have been in a position to look at current trends in infertility treatment from a very different perspective than their contemporaries. Being married, with children of her own, the elder one mixes regularly with mothers who are trying, with difficulty, to produce a sibling for their existing child, and it seems that infertility is the buzz-word, with conception problems being the trendiest life-style fashion of the day. When I was bringing up my children in the seventies, keeping up with the Joneses involved getting fitted carpets and taking a holiday on the Costa Lotta, but today's Joneses are all up to the limit on their credit cards after paying for treatment (ranging from hormone stimulation to full IVF procedures) at swish private fertility clinics. While both daughters have every sympathy for those who have conception difficulties, they are aware that there is a huge difference between treatment to help couples have their own babies and treatment with donated gametes to help couples give birth to other people's babies. Having experienced the joy of motherhood for herself, my elder daughter now views the prospect of egg donation with some alarm. She no longer visualizes the process as just giving away unneeded cells but as giving away her own children in the same way that babies are relinquished for adoption. Egg donorship would mean that there could be couples somewhere in the world with little replicas of her own two boys who would be growing up in an environment beyond her control, without ever knowing about her or their brothers. After much consideration my younger daughter, who loves children and has qualifications in childcare, has decided that if in the future she and a partner are unable to naturally conceive a genetically related baby, they will foster or adopt children. Failing that, they will get a dog. After experiencing infertility treatment from the other side of the fence, she is adamant that she would never choose to create a child through donated gametes.

Our grandchildren are still too young to appreciate any of the discussion on DI which has taken place around them, yet in some small way they have each demonstrated how important blood ties are to them. First, they both adore their father and seem to have a very special bond with him, delighting in playing with him and observing his every move with rapt admiration. They visibly thrive in his presence and share with him a unique relationship for which there can be no substitute. Three-year-old Daniel has shown an astute understanding of blood relationships and can explain in simple terms what a cousin is and why Uncle Matthew is a real uncle and why 'Uncle' Mark isn't. When his widowed paternal grand-mother remarried Daniel pedantically refused to call her new husband 'Grandad' because only Mummy's daddy and Daddy's daddy are Grandad. Baby Ryan has always had a particular fascination for his only blood grandfather. While other tots spout 'mum-mum' and 'da-da' as their first words, it was to my husband that he enthusiastically voiced his maiden utterance, 'Gan-dad!' At least for our grandchildren, we are the very people they believe us to be. For us as a family, DI has not had a destabilizing effect on our relationships and perceptions of each other, but it has shown us how self-interested decisions made by others in the past have impinged in a negative way on our lives. For me, my husband, and our heirs the reality of my missing ancestral heritage and incomplete medical history is something that we will have to continue to address in our own way, as and when circumstances demand.

Conversation between Caroline and Joanna (UK)

CL: Before you were told, did you ever think there was anything different about your family?

JR: Yes, I did. I remember when I was about six, cross-examining my mum (interestingly not my dad) about whether I was adopted or not. I remember asking her to promise me that she was really, really my mum and that Dad was really, really my dad. When I found out later on that wasn't the case, she justified it as saying, 'Well, he is your dad,' but I felt really angry that I had been lied to when I'd asked her to tell me the truth. Then in retrospect I didn't trust that she was my biological mother either.

CL: Why did you think that you might be adopted?

JR: I can't remember what triggered it at the time. I think I just thought it was a very important question to ask. I felt suspicious about it all, I don't remember exactly why. I just remember needing absolutely definite clarification on that issue.

CL: Why did your parents end up telling you the truth?

JR: My dad told me. I think he just thought it was something that needed to be told. What happened was that my dad had been crying and I asked what was the matter, and he said he couldn't tell me what was the matter, and I said, 'No, no, you have to tell me.' I thought I could cheer him up. So when he did tell me, my initial response was to wipe his tears away and give him a big kiss and a hug and say, 'You're the only dad I've got, the only dad I know. You're my dad and I love you.'

CL: Did you ever ask any questions?

JR: It wasn't really allowed. Because my dad was upset and I felt that I didn't want to upset him further. And my mum had told me that it was a family secret, just between the four of us. And my brother had told me not to make a fuss about it because it would drive my dad mad. The general impression was that I couldn't talk about it at all.

CL: You couldn't even talk to your brother about it?

JR: He pulled my hair at the time and said, 'Do you want to drive dad crazy? Shut up and don't make a fuss about it.' It wasn't done in the atmosphere of, 'Oh, I can go back and chat about this later.' It was serious.

I know that after I did get told I felt awful, but there was no one I could really go to because I'd been told by Mum that it was a family secret and that I mustn't tell anyone else. And I knew that if anyone saw me crying, I would get asked what the matter was. I was so upset because I wanted to cry and I didn't know where to cry.

So I ended up going into the school basement, which was a locker room, and I climbed up inside a chimney that had a big space where you could wedge yourself, and I cried there. But two kids came down into the basement and heard me crying, and they asked me what was wrong and I couldn't tell them, and then they went and got a teacher. She came down, and it all got terrible because I couldn't tell her, and I felt I was going to get into trouble for not telling what the matter was. It was just bloody awful. I can't remember what happened after that. All I remember was that it was getting worse and worse by the minute.

CL: What happened as you grew older?

JR: Later on, I bandied it around without understanding the meaning. It was strange. It was talked about within my family in a way, but there were barriers that you didn't go beyond. Like because Dad had written a book about it, you could say,

'AID.' It was talked about, but there was never a mention of the donor, so if I asked questions about why my skin was the colour it was, or why my skin wasn't the same colour as my brother's or my dad's, there was never any reply like, 'Because your donor is like this, or because his donor is like that.' It was always because I was more like one aunt and he was more like another. It was only when I was in my early twenties that I had any comprehension of another person being involved.

It was made clear to me that I would never get any information, and so it was something that was never to be pursued or discussed.

CL: When did you first realize the full significance of DI?

JR: The explanation of what it really meant, other than what it meant within my family, came after I had gone to live in Australia. I was invited to a conference to give a five-minute talk on donor insemination and what it meant for me. I didn't realize how little I had thought it all through, and I remember I just had a picture on a scrap of paper with all the different family members, and all I wanted to say was how different we all looked, and that I was very glad that I'd been told because I wouldn't have been able to make sense of it otherwise. I drew a picture of a light bulb to remind myself to 'keep it light.' Our family and our history aren't at all light, but I didn't feel it was necessary to expose that.

I remember afterwards people coming up to me and saying, 'But don't you want to meet your donor?' I remember initially saying, 'No,' and then going, 'Oh, oh, oh...' and my answer changed, and I think a few people realized that I was absolutely blown out and they arranged to meet me at a later date to talk things through, which was very lucky because it had just opened up the floodgates. All my fixed points of reference just disintegrated, my head was swimming. I had the most intense head-spin as all these thoughts whirled into my head that I had never been allowed to think about.

I had incredible dreams about it. It was just a complete opening up of things that there had been invisible walls around before.

CL: Have you found a similarity between your situation and that of adoptees that you've met?

JR: Definitely. I worked in Jigsaw,[1] and witnessed the pain of so many people who were trying to find out who their biological mothers and fathers are, and their other lost family members. I spoke at university about DI, and I had people come up to me afterwards, shaking and in tears – people who were conceived from affairs or from one-night stands, and who totally related to what I was saying. It's just a human response to a lack of information about ourselves and our families. Fostering, adoption, Stolen Generations,[2] affairs – whatever. It's a human response to something painful.

You just want to be understood. When you speak to adoptees, or to other people conceived by DI, or to somebody who just gets it, it's such a relief.

CL: Does your brother have similar thoughts to your own?

JR: He went through this at a different stage to me. He did it years before, and I didn't understand what he was talking about at that time, so we had quite a disagreement about it. He got in contact with the clinic and tried to get information. He said to me that it was so painful, and there were so many brick walls, and he banged his head against a brick wall for about ten years, and then he said he was exhausted and he was handing the baton on to me. But I know that if he could get answers, he still would.

CL: What have you done to find out information about your donor?

JR: What haven't I done? I've gone on the radio, I've gone on television, I've written to the guy who owned the clinic. I've spoken to people at the HFEA.[3] I've phoned all the government ministers I can get hold of. I'm trying to compile a human rights case to take to the European Court of Human Rights. I've gone to everybody and anybody I can think of for help. I've written to a donor from my clinic that I thought I was related to, and we had a gene test, which turned out to be negative. Since I realized how important it was, and what a big effect it was having on me, I've been trying and trying and trying.

CL: What thoughts have you got about why people don't want to help you?

JR: I've had different people say different things. Some people say that they understand and empathize, and say, 'Good luck.' Other people have vested interests and they don't want to help – like the doctors. Even with family members, I feel that they're protecting anybody other than me.

CL: Why do you think doctors don't want to help or change?

JR: I think it's a power issue. Because the clinics are powerful, and the doctors are powerful, and the industry's powerful, and the adults who want to conceive children and can't are powerful. They're a damn sight more powerful than people who haven't been conceived yet. I think it's just like it was with adoptees and members of the 'Stolen Generations'. It's going to well up at some stage, but it's going to take a lot of pain, and a lot of people to express that pain in a lot of ways, in order for it to be truly recognized. It's pretty tragic that people are making the same mistakes again.

CL: Should DI still go on or should it be different?

JR: To be honest, I don't think any parent should be encouraged to donate their genetic offspring. I don't think it's a good thing to foster in society – people giving away their children, or selling them for empathy, for money or for anything else. It's really a loaded question because in answering it, I know a lot of people will consequently disagree with everything else I have to say. But I don't think it is in the best interests of the child.

CL: Why do we think it's important to know our genetic history?

JR: It's normal in society. Look at the royal family in England. Worldwide, people have always had knowledge of where they come from, knowledge of their ancestors. It seems to be an innate part of our sense of humanity.

I don't think it's purely a psychological or a social thing, I think it's a spiritual thing. I can't even explain it. I'm working in Link-Up[4] with the 'Stolen Generations'. I'm going through file after file after file of different people who've felt this drive, and it seems to be just a natural reflex. It's important in society, and anybody who denies it is lying.

CL: How do you see your future?

JR: It's hard to look in the future, but initially when I started this, and when I turned to people and asked for help, I said things like, 'I'm only in my twenties and I don't have the energy to do all this, and I don't want to. I want to get on with my life.' I felt furious that I had been handed such a burden, and that I was expected to do something about it. I felt the energy of my youth was being drained by something that had been caused by the absolute negligence of a whole lot of people.

But gradually I'm coming to terms with the fact that that's the way it is. There are some people who are running with it, and I need to help them, just as they are helping me, and while I might have had nice ideas about doing other things with my life, it's very important that people understand what this is all about.

They're moving ahead without any qualms – debating the cloning of humans, for example. What kind of effect is that going to have on someone's identity? I just feel a responsibility to be involved with the people who are working for change, and also I think that lots of people who are working for change are really incredible people, and I think there's a real privilege in meeting those people.

CL: Do you think that some of your anger has been replaced by acceptance that there are certain things you won't be able to change?

JR: No, I'll never accept that. I remember one DI woman said to me that if she dies and she hasn't found out her information about her father and where she came from, she wants it written on her gravestone: 'She never found out, but she didn't go down without a fight.' I agree. I'll never give up. How can you just accept injustice and carry on with dignity?

Lots of people have said to me things like, 'Oh look, you're a pretty girl, Jo. You're intelligent, you've got a lot of things going for you, you've got a family that loves you – why don't you just get on with your life?' It's as if I had a large boulder on my leg that was causing me immense pain and suffering, and they just said to me, 'Oh don't worry about asking people to remove the boulder. Just saw your leg off, and hop around and have a good time.'

Barry (UK)

When I was conceived, there were good reasons for secrecy. In the UK masturbation was immoral. Sexual matters were not only private, they were shameful. Infertility was shameful, illegitimacy was utterly shameful. The practice of donor insemination was quasi-illegal, almost criminalized. We would have been bastards under law. The Church of England condemned it.

Things have changed, but secrecy is a legacy of that period. Secrecy is isolating, when you have a secret in a family, it is a barrier. When you have a secret, you have power over the person who does not know the secret. Many women feel the need to tell someone and kids tend to pick up on secrets. Plus, more and more and more families who are using assisted reproductive technology are telling their kids. They don't want to lie to them.

Secrecy and deception are ethically questionable, so secrecy obviously has serious problems. The father is especially isolated in DI, this is often not said.

And medically? You have to lie to a doctor when you are asked for your family medical history. No cancer, no heart disease, don't worry, you're not at risk. But you may be at risk. And this issue is only going to increase as genetics marches on. Most insurers, public or private, want to know if there is a family history of a disease, or whether the patient belongs to an ethnic group associated with the disease, before they will pay for a test. I had this experience myself with colonoscopy recently. So non-disclosure (secrecy) is hard to manage, it is not ethical, it damages the family, and when it comes to medical issues, there is no word for it but malpractice on the part of the doctor, and it is morally wrong on the part of the parents.

Once kids are told, I assure you, a large, large number will be curious about their origins. Just as adopted children have been curious about their origins.

We who seek to find our biological origins are told by the industry representatives and professionals that we don't need to know. How the hell do they know what it's like? We are supposed to demonstrate that harm has come to us, that there is some big wound deriving from a need to know in order to have access to information that almost everyone else takes for granted. Surely, the onus should be on those who wish to preserve secrecy to demonstrate why it should be preserved. Surely truth should be the default position, and deception that needs to be justified.

It is sometimes argued that because many people are deceived about who their father was (their mother had an extra-marital affair, for instance, and lied to her husband about the resulting child's origins), therefore, why should we need to know who our fathers were? Doctors who argue this routinely wildly exaggerate the percentage of people who are mistaken as to their paternity (some doctors claim 30%!), as an article in The Lancet a few years ago made clear; and as recent genetic work suggests, a mistaken paternity rate of perhaps less than 2 percent is common, excluding adopted kids who have been told. Do doctors really want to hold up adultery as the standard of care? But no matter, the argument is pathetic even if you accept its mistaken premise. It's like telling someone who has been robbed that they shouldn't worry because many other people have been robbed in the past and never got their property back. Or that it's OK to deliberately produce kids who are blind just because sometimes, tragically, kids are born blind by accident.

I resent the victim role one is pushed into playing in order to plead for what should be ours by right. Unless you can demonstrate some terrible wound, you shouldn't have the information, seems to be the attitude. And because DI kids seem fine, and are healthy on the surface, why rock the boat? This is very annoying. What we desire is what most people have as a matter of course. Knowledge of your origins. If your life story is a book, it's as though the first chapter is missing. Donor offspring have been deliberately deprived of key information, key to their medical needs (the absence of which can kill them) and key to their identity formation. Donor offspring express longing to know and great anger at these people who decided long ago to prevent us having knowledge.

I resent being told that genetic origin isn't important. Just look at all of our literature, our mythology. From Oedipus and Moses and King Arthur through Shakespeare and Dickens – Oliver Twist, the orphan, finding his biological family – up to Star Wars, 'Luke, I am your father.' Or if you scorn the arts, just look at the trend in the life sciences: it's all about the importance of DNA connections. The human genome project is a big deal. Why? Because we think that genes have a decided influence on our health, our personality and our behaviour. Suicide genes, risk-taking genes, coffee-loving genes.

The irony is that the reproductive medicine specialists are often the ones saying offspring don't need information on their origins, but the very science on which their craft is based is trumpeting more and more the importance of genetics. This, to put it kindly, is a contradiction. What it really is, is hypocrisy.

If it weren't, of course, for the importance of the genetic connection, mothers wouldn't seek DI. They'd just adopt. If it weren't for the importance of the genetic connection, doctors wouldn't provide donor sperm to women. They'd just recommend adoption. If it weren't for the importance of the genetic question, doctors wouldn't offer, and parents wouldn't ask for, the same donor when they go back for a second or third child. If it's important for them, why are they so surprised when it's important for us?

Let's look at the arguments in favour of preserving anonymity. First of all, the argument that donors will find themselves on the hook financially, it's a red herring. First, that's not what we want. But let's say some offspring does go for the family mansion of his donor. I doubt any court would even hear a case like that, but since this is a concern, all you have to do is just sever the rights and responsibilities of the donor in law and declare the social parents to be the parents. It ain't rocket science. Just like adoption and birth parents; nobody worries about adoptees going after their birth parents for money, do they? Why? Because there is a law. Britain, France, Sweden, Australia and most US states plus three provinces in Canada have produced legislation which states that the parents going through donor treatment are the only parents in law. Ontario has a law written, not just passed. It isn't a big deal. These laws completely protect gamete providers and recognize and honor the parents as those who chose to be the parents.

Second, there is the argument that donors would disappear if they knew that offspring might meet them one day. Again, complete crap. Sweden made identifiability upon maturity of the child the law 15 years ago. One state of Australia and the country of Austria have done similarly. New Zealand also stopped using anonymous donors. There are more sperm providers now available in New Zealand, despite the knee-jerk response from our opponents that they would all disappear. In fact, many, many semen providers who donated under the old, secret regime in NZ have expressed willingness and even interest in meeting offspring. The Sperm Bank of California, a non-profit organization, has been doing identity release for a while successfully; 80 percent of recipients want identity release donors, 75 percent of donors choose to be identifiable. Xytex, one of the biggest [sperm banks], in the US in Georgia is about to launch an identity release donor system.

Gamete donor anonymity makes it convenient for the clinic, and reduces the cost. Paying donors puts it on a commercial basis, which means you owe the donor nothing. There's a cost involved in using identifiable donors: tracking donors, tracking offspring, managing contact. So the biggest reason they argue for anonymity is really about cost and convenience. It's all about profit, kids.

I'm just from the first wave, the crudest turkey baster technology. The next wave, of IVF, are about 21. Egg donor offspring about ten years old maybe. And after them, possibly designer babies, when you start to manipulate the genes. There are already kids in New Jersey who have three biological parents. People who want to make money off of super athletes will likely be the first to start genetically modifying people. Bio-technology in the coming century is going to make the electronics revolution of the last couple of decades look like something going on in 'Toys R Us.' This is big business.

It's a very fundamental question. Are these people going to have the right to know how they were made, where they came from, to be afforded that dignity? Or are they going to be treated as products who don't need to know the ingredients that went into their production?

Put another way: can you manufacture people without ancestors? Is it just pre-modern crap that only the Amish or orthodox religious types care about ancestors? Or is there something meaningful and deeply necessary to being human in that connection to the past? In other words, is there something meaningful in our genetic connection to each other? Something sacred in fact, in the DNA?

The reason we haven't heard about this much yet is that most of us products of the industry are not yet old enough to make our voices heard. But if governments do nothing to open up this information, the new wave will make their voices heard. And they will be angry.

Nicky (UK)

To me, my life is a gift.

About DI, I do not feel bitter. I do not feel angry. I do not blame anyone. I do feel sad. I do wonder. I do contemplate my heritage, my biological history…my sense of continuity. I miss it. I'm not sure how being a DI offspring might have impacted on my life, apart from being aware that there is a whole side to myself I will never know about. A whole lineage…who are they, where are they?

I've had to forge a path on my own, discovering who I am, what I love and don't love, what my passion is or isn't, and finding the courage to pursue my truth. So, in one sense I have evolved without a reference point from one side of my heritage, which can be liberating on one hand and a hindrance on the other.

A hindrance because I do believe our character traits, aptitudes, sensibilities and talents can be passed on down through the generations and I feel as if I have been in conflict with these urges. I have not trusted them. Until now.

I have wondered whether the lack of a reference point (on my biological father's side) might have led to this protracted struggle to discover and validate myself. Relating to similar traits in your parents or relatives can be affirming for you. It can validate your interests and pursuits so you have more conviction in following them. I think I could have benefited from this.

I have had to let these natural urges push through me, revisit me, time and time again until I paid attention to their calling. And for the first time in my life, at 36 years old, I am determined to follow the career I love, not what I think I should be doing or could be doing…or being confused about what I want for myself. It's time to surrender to my heart and trust that life will take care of me.

I am not opposed to donor insemination, but I am opposed to secrets and lies in families, and to children not having access to information about their biological identity. It only leaves a gaping hole that is unfair and unnecessary…why burden someone with this kind of questioning or persistent curiosity!

In my case, I have a very loving family who have done the best they could with the little they knew about donor insemination. I have always felt loved and treasured by both my mother and (social) father. They answered my questions when I sensed that Dad wasn't my biological father and they have never resented me for or prevented me from, exploring the possibility of finding out information relating to my history. I respect and thank them for that.

I have had a wonderful life – so far – and I don't take it for granted. I'm grateful for it's mysteries, complexities, adventures, and opportunities.

What I would love to say to younger children who are conceived by donor sperm is – grasp your life, find the courage to be true to yourself, do what you love, and don't be afraid to reach out for help when you're in pain or struggling.

Between the family and friends I do have, I have found a profound sense of love, acceptance, and belonging. For me, there is nothing more precious.

Lynne (US)

When I was 35 years old, my father died of cancer. A few days later, my mother told both my sister and me that we were conceived through donor insemination. She said, 'Your father may not be your real father.' The timing was horrible, but I am glad to know the truth. I initially felt relief at the revelation, because it explained a lot of incongruities in my life. After researching DI, I became very troubled by it. The physicians did not allow me any information about the characteristics of my donor. I am still quite upset that I don't know half of my ethnic background. I also felt as if my foundation had been knocked out from under me. I find it sad that I never was able to talk to my dad about it. Instead of grieving for him, I was just so angry with him for lying to me about our relationship for all of our life together.

I never suspected DI in our family. My parents had told me that they had fertility problems and that the doctor had treated my mom so that they could have children. They just left off the rest of the story. I did know that my father had secrets from me. He would say things to me like, 'Little white lies are OK' and, 'Whatever you've been through, I've been through worse.' I knew that there were parts of himself which he did not share with us. When he was dying, my sister and I asked him what secrets he had, was there anything he wanted to talk to us about. He told us, 'It's none of your business.' So, despite his feeling that we were close, I did not share that belief. I knew that he was defended against us, and I knew that I could not talk with him about my true feelings.

The part of DI which has affected me the most is the secret nature of it. I feel that if there is nothing wrong with creating children in this way, then there is no need for secrecy. Secrecy implies that the procedure is shameful, that I am shameful, that there is something wrong with me. Indeed, I don't have the full rights of most human beings to know my true identity and my real roots. This pains me deeply. Not knowing who my genetic father is and being denied information about him is like having a broken heart that won't heal. I feel like I should be grateful to have been given life, yet it feels like an incomplete life, and the pain of being denied my full self sometimes outweighs the benefit of having part of a life.

Trust is also a major issue for me. Even before I knew of my DI origins, I had figured out that I grew up having to rely on myself and take care of my own needs emotionally. Feelings weren't acceptable in my family. In my family, if I didn't have a smile on my face, my father would ask in a panic, 'Are you OK?' I had to say yes to keep him together. I think my lack of trust developed long before I knew of my DI origins. The little white lies and the distance between us led me to develop independently, not wanting to rely on others for support. I have worked on this issue a lot in my life, but I still have difficulty with intimate relationships, just being myself (or knowing who I am for that matter) and feeling free to expose myself to others.

I do believe that DI should be allowed to continue, but with some caveats. Most important, I believe it essential that the people born from DI be able to know the truth of their lives from the beginning. They should know the truth of the relationships in their life, have as much information as possible about all three of their parents, and be able to meet their sperm donor. I believe that the more accepting the parents are of the procedure, or the relationships, and of the child, the better the child will feel about themselves. The individual conceived through DI deserves to be accepted for who they are, their true nature, interests, and temperaments.

I also firmly believe that there needs to be legislation about DI, including records kept of genetic links, and monitored limitations on how many offspring each donor can conceive.

Lauren (Australia)

I was told about my conception when I was nine years old. My parents had been agonizing over it for years and they decided they would tell us before my older brother started high school. They sat us down one afternoon and told us how special we were and that they loved us very much. They explained to my brother and me how our father wasn't our biological father and Mum had visited a doctor to be inseminated with an anonymous man's sperm.

At the time I wasn't interested. I think while they were talking we were staring impatiently out the window, keen to go outside and play with our friends. Afterwards we hugged our parents and told them we loved them very much.

I never suspected that I wasn't my father's child. However, according to Mum, they sat us down and said, 'We have something important to tell you...' and my brother replied, 'I'm adopted, aren't I?' They were extremely shocked. But, luckily, they persevered and shared their secret with us.

I think it just goes to show that children are very perceptive. They can sense when things aren't right, especially when, as was my brother's case, they don't look like the rest of the family. Also, I believe it is not what DI and adoptive parents say to their children but it is what they don't say. My parents never said, 'You look so much like your father' or, 'You have the same personality as your Nana.' Subconsciously, my brother picked up on this, and his doubts grew until they led to the most obvious conclusion – adoption. But, however, adoption still didn't explain my appearance; one of his most vivid memories is going in to the hospital to visit Mum after my birth.

I believe that we need procedures like DI and IVF; I really feel for people who are unable to realize their dreams of having children. However, many changes need to be made to these procedures. Doctors need to be made more accountable for their actions.

The rights of the children must be made paramount in assisted reproductive technologies. We didn't have any choices in the beginning – we were simply created and I think people forgot we would grow into intelligent adults. I believe we should have the choice to access our birth information, if that is what we desire. I wish I was at least given that choice.

Janice (UK)

My story begins a long time ago, but it is one that I share with others, perhaps many hundreds of others. Our origin was forever to be a secret. Many of us are in the dark about our beginning, but we don't know it; only a few of us know the truth, and I am one of them. Our parents were told never to tell. Most of us are walking around believing that we are the offspring of the two parents who brought us up. But there is a twist to our story. We are only biologically related to our mother. The man listed as 'father' on our birth certificates is the man who raised us, but he is not our biological father. Our fathers' identity remains a mystery. We were never to know the truth. The truth was too terrifying a burden to place on children who were born of such an unorthodox procedure, seen as from the world of science fiction. But then a few of us found out, some of us were told, and we want to tell our stories.

I belong to a group of people who are 'donor offspring,' those conceived via artificial insemination from an anonymous sperm donor. In England, in the late 1940s, my parents, faced with infertility, sought help from a pioneering London gynaecologist, Mary Barton. Then, she was one of only two physicians who were brave enough to experiment with donor insemination (DI) in aiding infertile couples to conceive and give birth to the children they so badly wanted. The carefully orchestrated procedure was not only successful in determining my own conception, but also was responsible for the birth of my brother, four-and-a-half years later.

In contrast to some other reports of families with donor offspring, ours was a relatively uneventful childhood. Overtly, we were not aware of the fact that the truth was being withheld from us. My parents had been advised not to tell, and they kept their agreement. We never suspected that we were not like every other family we knew. Friends and relatives cooed over us as children and even commented on how much we resembled our father and our mother.

Disclosure came when I was 22 and my brother 18, six months after the death of my father. Our mother carefully and lovingly told us the truth of our origin. Though originally loyal to our father's desire that we should never know of his infertility, and of the choice of DI, she felt that we should know the truth after all. It was an immense surprise and shock. I remember examining my hands and face in the mirror, seeking physical evidence of this 'new' biological father's presence, being fascinated by the prospect that half of me was 'unknown.' I also felt sadness and frustration that I would never be able to talk about this new revelation about my identity with the man whom I had now discovered was my 'social' father; but he was still my 'father.' I wanted to tell him how I admired him and my mother for the courage that it took to choose DI, when the Church and even the medical profession had looked upon this procedure with vitriol. I wanted to tell him that I was glad to be alive.

Years passed and I followed the path life presented to me, moving to the US, obtaining a graduate degree in social work, working, marrying and giving birth to a daughter. I had somehow incorporated the meaning of this 'new' part of me and had grown to accept my birth origin. I thought about it very little.

Things gradually changed when my daughter was to reach the age of majority. My 'job' as a parent was shifting and, as many do approaching middle age, I began to re-examine who I was, what was important to me, and where I was in my life. One-half of my biological origin was still a mystery, and my daughter was about to start her life as an adult, still not being able to identify one quarter of her own biological background. What genes do we carry that may be associated with disease? Am I a woman who carries the BRCA1 gene? Women from Ashkenazi Jewish families are more likely than other women to carry this gene that causes an increase in the risk of breast cancer. Was my donor father Jewish? It became important to me as a person, and as a parent to my daughter, to discover more.

My quest began a little over a year ago, and what an amazing, intense experience it has been. The Internet has been an invaluable tool. It has allowed me to communicate with others involved who live from one end of the globe to the other. I have been amazed at how incredibly open individuals have been in sharing such personal, detailed stories of their own. Some stories have been poignant and sad; others more joyful. Why do I want to know who my father was? I have come to realize that every person has a need to know. To know one's family history, to know where one fits, to which group one belongs, both to feel valued as an individual but also to feel part of a group.

These encounters have forced me to ask fundamental questions of myself. How comfortable am I admitting to others that I am the offspring of an unknown sperm donor? Do I feel a stigma? Did I choose my 'helping' profession because, at an unconscious level, I wanted to resolve my own personal issues around being a donor offspring? Or, as someone who is relatively healthy and stable as a person, was I wanting to reach out to help others who are less able, struggling with their own issues of identity?

Why do I want to know who my donor father was? Who will my donor father be, if he still lives? He is a man about whom I am immensely curious. Is he a person who has been happy with his life? Has he pursued a professional career, as I have? Is he creatively talented and did he gravitate towards the arts in his life, as I have? What made him laugh and gave him pleasure? Would he be proud of the offspring he created? Was he a parent to children he raised who are half-siblings of mine? Would he like to meet me, and would he be pleased to know that he contributed to making me the person that I am?

The fact that a British journalist was preparing a television documentary on the history of artificial insemination in England (Witness: Secret Fathers) led me to hear of another offspring conceived at Mary Barton's clinic, besides my brother and me. I happened to be in England on holiday when the program was aired, and was both nervous and fascinated to meet him. Though strangers to each other, we comfortably talked openly about the unidentified sperm that contributed to our existence and the feelings we had upon first being told that a 'turkey baster' had helped give us life. The meeting was profound, and I wanted him to meet my brother. Strangely enough, a month to the day after this first encounter, the three of us were together. We had begun to brainstorm the idea that a website might be set up where DNA profiles of donor off-spring could be posted. People might find half-siblings, and perhaps through this, their donor fathers. We three sent in our blood samples for DNA testing to begin the process.

The results of the DNA testing were a revelation: I was overjoyed to find out that I am indeed a 'full' sibling of my brother, even though he was conceived four-and-a-half years after me. But imagine my utter amazement and incredulity to discover that both of us are half-siblings of the only other man that we knew to have been conceived at Mary Barton's clinic! We all three share the same donor father! The odds of making this discovery must be infinitesimal. They also suggest that the clinic donor pool was pretty small. It is a disquieting fact that back then, some champion donors contributed to the births of over one hundred children. So, how many other half-siblings do we have? We will never know the answer to that question. Do I want to meet and get to know half-siblings? Yes. Most of us are ignorant of the fact that we are not the sons and daughters of the father listed on our birth certificates. But for the few of us, who do know, perhaps some of us may find each other; and some of us may even find out more about our donor fathers.

I have evolved to a place where it is important to me to continue my 'quest.' The story is still on going. I do not know my donor father's identity and may never know. But I am enjoying getting to know our 'new' half-sibling and I want to keep in contact with others involved in the issue. I keep adding to my 'stork file' as each new piece of the puzzle falls into place. I know that some parts of it may never be finished. But I'm willing to be open to wherever the quest takes me. In the meantime, I feel secure in myself, and am profoundly glad of the fact that my parents gave me life and that I am here.

Notes

1   Post-adoption resource centre in Queensland, Australia. Jigsaw works with adoptees and their families (natural and adoptive), providing counseling, support, and assistance with tracing.

2   From the early 1900s to the mid 1970s, the policy of successive Australian Governments towards Aboriginal and Torres Strait Islander people was to systematically destroy their identity and culture. They tried to achieve this by forcibly removing thousands of Aboriginal and Torres Strait Islander people's babies and small children, taking them from their families and communities, and then arranging for

them to be brought up within White culture. This either meant that they went to White families (adoption or fostering) or White institutions (children's homes or juvenile detention centres). The men and women who were abducted in this way are the Stolen Generations.

3   The Human Fertilisation and Embryology Authority in the UK. The HFEA was set up in 1991 as the regulatory body for the fertility industry in the UK. They also hold the records for everyone who was created by assisted reproductive techniques in the UK from 1991 onwards, including full information about their genetic identity.

4   Link-Up (Queensland) Aboriginal Corporation. This is the Queensland branch of Link-Up, which is a national resource centre for Aboriginal and Torres Strait Islander people. Link-up works to reunite the Stolen Generations with their natural families, and provides counseling and support. Link-Up also runs programs to educate and inform the general public about the Stolen Generations.

Glossary

AI
Artificial insemination, see donor insemination.

AIH
Artificial insemination by husband.

Azoospermia
The absence of sperm in the semen.

Clomiphene (or Clomid)
A drug used to stimulate ovulation.

DC
Donor conception, including all forms of conception using donated reproductive tissue, donor insemination, donor egg, and donor embryo.

DI
Donor insemination. The use of sperm from a donor which is placed in the cervix or uterus of a woman.

Donor embryo
Embryos formed during IVF which are not used after a couple completes their family may be donated to another infertile couple.

Egg donation (also called donor oocyte)
Eggs provided by a donor who has been stimulated with hormones to produce a number of eggs.

Epididymis
A structure where sperm collects on the way to the vas deferens.

Gametes
Sperm or eggs that are used to create an embryo.

GIFT
Gamete intra-fallopian transfer. The placing of an egg and sperm in the fallopian tubes where they will hopefully fertilize naturally.

ICSI
Intracytoplasmic injection. The injecting of a single sperm into an egg in order to fertilize it.

Implantation
When an embryo beds itself into the wall of the uterus.

IVF
In vitro fertilization. An egg and sperm are fertilized in a glass dish and then when the cells have divided the resulting embryo is transferred into the woman's uterus.

Laparoscopy
Surgical procedure where a small telescopic device is inserted into a woman's abdomen in order to look at the pelvic organs.

Motility
The forward movement of the sperm.

Varicocele
Dilation of veins in the cord down which sperm travels.

Vas deferens
The tube which takes the sperm from the epididymis to the urethra (and which carries the urine and ejaculate to outside the body).

Suggested Reading

Friedman, J.S. (1997) *Building your Family through Egg Donation*. Fort Thomas, KY: Jolance Publishing.
This book looks at the emotional impact of egg donation and what to tell the children.

Snowden, R. and E. (1993 revised) *Gift of a Child*. Exeter: University of Exeter Press.
Non-technical information about childlessness caused by male infertility and the use of DI. Also includes information on the UK Human Fertilization and Embryology Act (1990).

Noble, E. (1987) *Having your Baby by Donor Insemination*. Boston: Houghton Mifflin.
Noble used a known donor to conceive her child. She looks at the practical, legal and ethical problems faced by infertile couples who are thinking about using donor conception.

Frost-Vercollone, C., and Moss, R. and H. (1997) *Helping the Stork*. London: MacMillan.
Written by two social workers and a psychologist. The Mosses have two DI children. Looks at some of the choices and challenges of DI.

Lorbach, C. (ed) (1997) *Let the Offspring Speak*. Available from the Donor Conception Support Group of Australia (see Useful Contacts list).
This book is a collection of the papers presented at the first consumer-hosted conference dealing with donor conception. It also includes short articles written by a number of adults born by donor conception.

Baran, A and Pannor, R. (1989) *Lethal Secrets*. New York: HarperTrade.
The psychology of donor insemination. Discusses the emotional implications of keeping secrets in DI families.

Gordon, E. R. (1992) *Mommy Did I Grow in Your Tummy?* Santa Monica, CA: EM Greenberg Press.

An illustrated book aimed at four to eight year age group. Briefly describes the concepts of IVF, sperm donation, egg donation, surrogacy, and adoption.

Infertility Research Trust (1991) *My Story.* Infertility Research Trust.

Designed to aid in telling young children (from approx. three to eight years old) about being born by donor insemination. It contains colourful, simply drawn pictures. Available through the Donor Conception Network (see Useful Contacts list).

Carter, J. W. and M. (1997) *Sweet Grapes – How to stop being infertile and start living again.* Indianapolis: Perspectives Press.

'When you are chasing the dream of a baby it is easy to forget that life has the potential for many other dreams and fulfilments.'

Moyle, P. (1990) *Where did I come from?* New York: Carol Publishing Group.

A book that explains the process of reproduction simply and with illustrations that children will like.

Useful Contacts

Donor conception support groups

Donor Conception Support Group of Australia Inc.

PO Box 53
Georges Hall
NSW 2147
Australia

Web page: www.members.optushome.com.au/dcsg
Email: dcsg@optushome.com.au
Telephone: +61 (2)9724 1366

This international group started in 1993 helps to meet the needs of: families with donor children; people considering using or currently on donor sperm; egg or embryo programs; adults conceived by donated gametes; donors past and present; and anyone interested in donor issues. The group has published a book, *Let the Offspring Speak* (see Suggested Reading) with articles by offspring, parents, donors, and many others. It currently publishes two leaflets: *Where did I come from?* for older donor offspring and *Not my Child* for potential donors. The group advocates for legislation in the area of donor conception in many countries and also for the right of donor offspring to have access to donor information.

The New Reproductive Alternatives Society

Email: spratten@nisa.et

This is Canada's first support group for DI families (formed in 1987). They are also a national lobby group which has worked for years with government, policy makers, and the media, trying to bring about reform so that the system serves the needs of the offspring as a priority.

The Donor Conception Network

PO Box 265
Sheffield
S3 7YX
UK

Web page: www.dcnetwork.org
Email: dcnetwork@appleonline.net
Telephone: +44 (0)208 245 4369

This organization is a family-to-family support network for those who have founded their families with the aid of donated gametes (eggs, sperm, and embryos) and for those considering doing so. It is also an educational resource for professionals and the general public on the long-term implications of using donated gametes. The network publishes a series of leaflets about donor conception.

ACeBabes

8 Yarwell Close
Derwent Heights
Derby
DE21 4SW
UK

Web page: www.acebabes.co.uk
Email: enq@acebabes.co.uk
Telephone: +44 (0)1332 832558

This is a network of parents who have been successful after assisted conception. The group aims to support parents through the early days of pregnancy into family life. There are specific issues which they have to face: the large number of multiple pregnancies; dealing with frozen embryos; trying for siblings or deciding to end treatment; telling children about their conception whether or nor donor gametes have been used. The group continues to support families as the children become older and want to find out more or speak to others conceived the same way.

Donor conception websites and bulletin boards

www.groups.yahoo.com/group/SpermDonors/

This internet discussion group looks at issues of known versus unknown donation. It was created by a former donor. The discussion archives are publicly available and include postings from donors, offspring, parents, those considering treatment, and other interested people.

www.PCVAI@yahoo.com

The title of this website is short for 'people conceived via artificial insemination.' This group is restricted to DI adults and teens so that they can be confident about not having to deal with others criticizing their feelings. DI adults may join by visiting the website and following the instructions to send an email to the moderators.

www.DonorsOffspring.com

An online database and bulletin board begun by Greg Wiatt. It was created for those in search of siblings conceived through donor insemination and donors.

General infertility support groups

European Infertility Network

Woodlawn House
Carrickfergus
Co. Antrim
Northern Ireland
BT3 8PX

Web page: www.ein.org
Email: webmaster@ein.org
Telephone: +44 (0)7885 138101

Aims to provide quality up to date information and news on Assisted Human Reproduction, infertility, getting pregnant and other apsects of infertility information. It also wishes to stimulate infertility information dissemination among professionals, researchers and patients in the area of Infertility.

Resolve: The National Infertility Association

1310 Broadway
Somerville
MA 02144
USA

Web page: www.resolve.org
Email: info@resolve.org
Telephone: 888 623 0744

A nationwide organization, split into local chapters. It is dedicated to providing education, advocacy and support to men and women facing infertility. It provides a helpline, physician referral services and member to member contact system and publications on infertility.

The American Infertility Association

666 Fifth Avenue
Suite 278
New York
NY 10103

USA

Web page: www.americaninfertility.org
Email: info@americaninfertility.org
Telephone: 718 621 5083

The mission of this national organization is to serve as a lifetime resource for men and women needing reproductive information and support and to forward the causes of adoption and reproductive health through advocacy, education, awareness building and research funding. It provides support groups in the New York area, infertility reference libraries, free seminars on infertility treatment, a monthly newsletter and a telephone peer support network.

The Infertility Network

160 Pickering Street
Toronto
ON
M4E 3J7
Canada

Web page: www.InfertilityNetwork.org
Email: Info@InfertilityNetwork.org
Telephone: (1) 416 691 3611; Fax (1) 416 690 8015

This independent, charitable organization provides information, support, and referrals; seminars (live and on tape/CD); support groups; an email newsletter; and bi-annual mailings on topics related to infertility, donor conception, and adoption, as well as on reproductive and genetic technologies.

CHILD

Charter House
43 St Leonards Road
Bexhill on Sea
East Sussex
TN40 1JA
UK

Web page: www.child.org.uk
Email: office@email2.child.org.uk
Telephone: +44 (0)1424 732 361

The national infertility patient support network in the UK offering a 24-hour telephone service; helpline; regional support groups; medical advisers; quarterly magazine, CHILDchat; fact sheets; information days. CHILD's mission is to provide high-quality information and support to those suffering from infertility and to promote public awareness of infertility and its impact on people's quality of life.

IFIPA (International Federation of Infertility Patient Associations)

Contact details: as for CHILD.

Formed in 1993 this organization currently comprises 16 national fertility patient associations representing 12 different countries. The mission of IFIPA is to unite and support infertility patient organizations around the world. It is committed to educating and promoting infertility awareness and the needs and concerns of infertile people in the medical, scientific, and political arenas. IFIPA provides a global perspective on the problems faced by infertile people and the options available to them.

ACCESS

PO Box 959
Parramatta
NSW 2124
Australia

Web page: www.access.org.au
Email: info@access.org.au
Telephone: +61 (2) 9670 2380

This group, based in Australia, is a consumer-based organization which provides support, education, and advocacy for infertile people. Member services include a range of 38 fact sheets, a newsletter and the OPTIONS group which provides contact for people who share similar infertility experiences such as: options for men; approaching life without children; donor options; and options after IVF miscarriage.

Fertility New Zealand

PO Box 34 151
Birkenhead
Auckland
New Zealand

Web page: www.fertilitynz.org.nz
Email: nz.infertility@clear.net.nz

This is the national organization for those affected by infertility. It is a non-profit consumer-based organization committed to promoting the well-being and welfare of all people affected by infertility through representation in the general community and the medical, scientific, and political arena. They have local branches and offer information support networking and advocacy.

IDI (Information donogene Insemination)

Heidenfarht 23b
55262 Heidesheim
Germany

Website: www.wunschkind.de (see link: IDI)
Email: sven.williamson@t-online.de
Telephone: +49 (0)6132 56343

This is the only self-help group operating in Germany. Its website can found as a subsite of the one above.

Counseling and social work groups

PROGAR (The Project Group on Assisted Reproduction of the British Association of Social Workers)

51a Great King Street
Edinburgh
EH3 6RP
Scotland

Email: e.d.blyth@hud.ac.uk
Telephone: +44 (0)1865 553685

This group focuses attention on the needs of those personally involved in assisted conception: individuals born as a result of treatment, donors and their children, recipients, and prospective parents.

BICA (British Infertility Counsellors Association)

69 Division Street
Sheffield
S1 4GE
UK

Web page: www.bica.net
Telephone helpline: +44 (0)1342 843880

This group aims to encourage and facilitate its members to provide the highest standards of counselling support to people affected by fertility issues. It publishes the *Journal of Infertility Counselling* three times a year.

Australian and New Zealand Infertility Counselors Association (ANZICA)

The Secretary
c/o Reproductive Medicine Unit
The Queen Elizabeth Hospital
Woodville Road
Woodville
SA 5011
Australia

Email: Lofty@arcom.com.au

The aim of ANZICA is to represent the interests of infertility counsellors and to provide a forum for the exchange of ideas, mutual support, and training.

Index